TAKING CHARGE
OF
FIGHTING CANCER

an easy to use workbook

Stephanie R. Carter, Ph.D.

iUniverse, Inc.
Bloomington

Taking Charge of Fighting Cancer
an easy to use workbook

Copyright © 2011 Stephanie R. Carter, Ph.D.

The information, ideas, and suggestions in this book are not intended as a substitute for professional medical advice. Before following any suggestions contained in this book, you should consult your personal physician. Neither the author nor the publisher shall be liable or responsible for any loss or damage allegedly arising as a consequence of your use or application of any information or suggestions in this book.

iUniverse books may be ordered through booksellers or by contacting:

iUniverse
1663 Liberty Drive
Bloomington, IN 47403
www.iuniverse.com
1-800-Authors (1-800-288-4677)

Because of the dynamic nature of the Internet, any Web addresses or links contained in this book may have changed since publication and may no longer be valid. The views expressed in this work are solely those of the author and do not necessarily reflect the views of the publisher, and the publisher hereby disclaims any responsibility for them.

Any people depicted in stock imagery provided by Thinkstock are models, and such images are being used for illustrative purposes only.

Certain stock imagery © Thinkstock.

ISBN: 978-1-4620-1377-7 (pbk)
ISBN: 978-1-4620-1378-4 (ebk)

Printed in the United States of America

iUniverse rev. date: 5/11/2011

For all my patients who shared their healing journeys with me.
And for Linda and Myrna.

Acknowledgements

This book is a product of many years treating people with cancer. I am eternally grateful for all that my patients shared with me and for all that they taught me. To say that it has been my great privilege to work with them through their fight for life, and for some, their dying and death, is an understatement. They have enriched my life and given me gifts that I hope I'm able to pass on to others. By writing this book, I am thanking them all.

To my friends and colleagues: Thank you to Barbara, Carolyn, Camilla, Greg, and Peggy, for reading the manuscript and for your words of encouragement; to Holly, for not only reading, encouraging and telling me how I must get this book out, but for all that listening; to Debbie, whose editing skills appear on many pages; to the Powerful Mind group at the Cancer Support Community of Greater Miami who sat with me and experienced the CD and gave me their feedback. To all of you, my gratitude and thanks.

To my family: To Jon and Alex, thank you for your reading and helpful comments and especially for your constant encouragement. To Nicole and Dana, thank you for your interest. To Francis, my dear husband and partner in life, thank you for your deep belief that I can do anything, your help every step of the way, and of course, for your superb editing skills.

To all of my dear ones, I love you, I'm proud of you and you do great things every day.

Contents

Personal Introduction

Looking back, I first began thinking about this book in 1963. That was the year one of my best friends, Linda, was diagnosed with cancer. She died many months later. I was 16 years old. I think she was 17 years old by the time she died. We spent a lot of time together both through her brave fight for life and then during the time she knew she would die. I remember so much. I remember our many conversations about life and death, about her fears and her pain, about her joys and sorrows, but mostly, I remember how she came to understand love in a way that has taken me many years to learn.

I also remember how we needed help. We needed help in understanding what was happening to her and help in understanding what was happening to me. But there wasn't any. Neither of our parents knew to get psychological help for us. We didn't know of any books to read. So, we two teenagers listened to each other and did the best we could.

I listened and watched as she used the power of her mind. I was amazed at her outlook on life, awed by her determination, attitude, and strong will. At the time, I sensed that she gave herself extra time and certainly a better quality of life because of these strengths. I think that if she had access to all the cancer treatments that are available today, along with the power of her positive and wise mind, she would have survived the cancer.

She left me wondering what it was all about. What was this powerful mind/body/spirit interaction that I witnessed in her? What was that strength she was drawing from that enabled her to stay connected to me, other friends, and family, live longer, and smile up until the very end?

Not surprisingly, my experience with my dear friend was a powerful influence in my choice to study psychology. I started working with children and their families, and I quickly learned that the differences in people's lives is not always what happens to them, but how they interpret what happens to them. People who talk to themselves in positive ways feel better about their lives. People who talk to themselves in negative ways are not so happy. Over time, I noticed the interaction of mind and body. The children and families who worked at keeping a positive mental attitude seemed to get sick less, solved problems more quickly, seemed to be generally more satisfied with their lives. They felt more in control, even though the same difficulties were happening to them.

I began to wonder about meditation. In 1974, I read *How to Meditate, A Guide to Self-Discovery* by Lawrence Le Shan. My husband and I began to meditate, and discovered how calmed and in control we felt. Even when our lives were chaotic, we felt calm and centered.

In 1981, I found Norman Cousin's *Anatomy of an Illness* at the bookstore and read his story about how he used the power of his mind to overcome a serious illness. I remember my excitement about the concept of mind/body healing. Within the month, I developed a serious autoimmune problem which doctors could not diagnose. I was in terrible pain and felt like I would die. But, I didn't feel out of control. I felt blessed that I had read Norman Cousin's book, and immediately adopted his plan for keeping my mood positive as I imagined myself recovered. I recovered eventually, and I believe that the illness was less traumatic for me because I felt I had control over myself and my healing.

Other life events happened to me, my family, my friends, and my patients, that influenced me to explore the connections among mind, body, and spirit. I watched people's minds help their bodies feel better and recover from a variety of problems. I watched as people's bodies challenged their minds to learn something new and helpful. And I watched people learning about love, connecting to others, and about being the best person they could be as their spiritual selves emerged.

Along the way, I learned about using visual imagery for healing. That was another blessing. In 1992 I had pneumonia. It came on quickly and it was a deadly kind. My doctor told me that the antibiotics were not working and that I might die. Again, I felt blessed that I knew about the power of my mind. I went into a meditative state and imagined my immune system hard at work in and around my lungs, and I imagined myself well. Within 24 hours the pneumonia was in retreat, and I made a quick recovery. I believe that I was able to mobilize my immune system by using the power of my mind so that the antibiotics could start working. In my meditation, I felt I became one with the Universe and connected to peace. Using the power of my mind and spirit along with the power of modern medicine was the combination I needed to live.

I have witnessed what happened to me, happen to others. I have been privileged to witness friends and patients recover from illness by using the power of their minds to connect mind, body and spirit for healing. I have been privileged to be with people who have prolonged their lives, who have created a precious quality of life, and who discovered that living through serious illness brings special learning, wisdom, and love.

I'm still working on what happened to Linda and me. Linda moved on in spirit and I moved on in life. Her life and death were an exquisite gift to me. She started me on a journey of connection, of finding the balance in mind, body, and spirit. She opened the door to my knowing that I can sit with other people's pain, and that I can sit with my own. She taught me that I can be with people in a positive, healing way. She taught me that I am happy when I'm learning, and happiest when I pass that learning on. I hope I can pass on to you the learning that began with my childhood friendship with Linda.

Introduction:
About the Workbook

Since you are reading this, it's likely that you or someone you care about has been diagnosed with cancer. Although this can be frightening and your thoughts may be turning toward mortality, I'd like to help you feel calmer and less vulnerable *and* improve your chances to fight the cancer. With so many advances in detection and treatment, the prognosis for recovery keeps getting better and better.

As you may know, patients who are actively involved in the treatment of their disease not only feel more in control, but also have better outcomes. Dr. George Solomon and Dr. Lydia Temoshok, researchers in the field of psychoneuroimmunology (the study of the interaction of the mind, immune and neurological systems, or "mind/body interactions"), have identified the following characteristics among long-term survivors of cancer.

- They are realistic and accept their diagnosis, but they don't take it as a death sentence.
- They have a fighting spirit and they learn how not to be helpless or hopeless.
- They work to change their lifestyles.
- They learn how to handle stress effectively.
- They are aware of their psychological and physical needs, and they take care of them.
- They talk openly about their illness.
- They take personal responsibility for their health, and they consider their treating physicians as team members.
- In whatever ways they can, they help other people with cancer.

I have created the CD *Fighting Cancer* and this workbook in order to guide you in developing these characteristics. *This is a "how-to" book.* I will show you *how to* do the things you need to do in order to develop the characteristics of long-term survivors of cancer. You'll learn how to take care of yourself in body, mind, and spirit. I know that you already are working toward developing these characteristics because you are reading this book and listening to the CD. You can have all of them. *I'll show you how.*

In **Taking Charge 1**, you'll learn to be your own first priority and put yourself first. You'll learn about the CD, your immune system, and more. In the first chapter *I show you how to* do visual imagery. Visual imagery is an important tool in cancer recovery because it creates a connection between your body, mind, and spirit. It helps you manage stress better, calms your body, activates your immune system, reduces pain, and makes you feel better. You clear your mind. It enhances your healing, calms your mind, and connects you to your personal spiritual beliefs. You'll feel more in control of yourself. You will learn how to motivate yourself and imagine yourself well. You will practice success and achieve success.

In **Taking Charge 2**, you'll learn about the feelings that you're experiencing now. *I show you how to* identify your feelings. I give you a chart of emotional and physical feelings that will help you sort it all out. This is important because your feelings give you a wealth of important information. If you don't know what your feelings are then they won't be useful. It is vital for you to be able to express how you feel so that you can talk about what is happening to you, so that you can use the appropriate strategy to feel better, so that you can be a better reporter to your healthcare providers about what you are feeling in body, mind, and spirit. Then, they can do a better job for you.

In **Taking Charge 3**, you'll learn about Integrative Cancer Care and how to use it. Integrative Cancer Care includes medical, complementary, and alternative care. *I show you how to* be the Captain of your team and ask the right questions to get the information you need to make the best decisions for yourself.

In **Taking Charge 4**, you'll learn about creating an even more powerful mind. *I show you how to* change your negative thinking patterns into positive ones. You learn hope, focused determination, a good attitude, and how to use your strong will. Cancer survivors believe that their ability to maintain a positive, hopeful attitude increases their chances for recovery, and research suggests that they are right.

In **Taking Charge 5**, you'll learn about connections. *I show you how to* connect with people, communicate with the important people in your life, and use social support. Research has shown that cancer patients who use social support live longer. Cancer survivors can tell you how connecting to others enriched the quality of their lives.

In **Taking Charge 6**, you'll learn about spirituality. *I show you how to* explore your own personal beliefs and make them a part of your life now. Spirituality is a special kind of connection and support that people find in different ways. Some people find their spirituality through their religion, others through a different belief system, and others by being the best person they can be. Cancer patients commonly rely on spirituality and religion to help them cope with the cancer and the effects it has on their lives. There is evidence that spirituality can have a positive impact on health. It provides comfort, hope, and healing.

In **Taking Charge 7**, you'll learn about managing your time. *I show you how to* organize yourself so that you can do everything necessary to achieve wellness. At times, all that you have to do will feel overwhelming. Breaking down your goals and tasks into a doable daily diary will help you feel calmer and more in control. You'll take comfort in knowing that you are taking good care of yourself.

The information in this workbook is what I talk about with my patients who are fighting cancer. I strongly urge everyone to start immediately with the *Fighting Cancer* CD. Right away, they feel comforted and calmer.

Everyone talks about these issues at their own pace, and in the order that they need. That's why I have designed this workbook to be used in any order. You can go to the sections that you need first and read those, or you can read through in the order presented.

The workbook exercises can also be done in any order. You'll find that as you go through the phases of your treatment your answers may change. Even the names of your healthcare providers may change. Your goals may change. What you want and desire may change. You will experience emotional, physical, and spiritual changes on this journey and experience a growth that is hard to imagine now.

I think of this workbook as a moving circle, like a wheel. In the center is your self, or what I think of as the soul. Connected in all directions are your body, mind, and spirit. The better the balance among the three, the easier the wheel rolls and you get to where you want to be.

Every one of us is a circle with our selves at the center. We are our minds, our bodies, and our spirits. They are inter-connected, not separate. We just separate them in order to think about them. In order to take care of ourselves, our souls, we have to learn how to take the best care of these three parts of ourselves. This is especially important for you, now that you are fighting against cancer and fighting for life. This is your primary task.

Each point on the circle – the mind, the body, the spirit - represents some aspect of wisdom or something to contemplate. Each point is a way of learning what we need to know to heal our souls. Your way may first be through your body as you get medical treatment and work on diet, exercise, and get massages. Other people might use their minds first, learning positive thinking skills. Others might turn to spirituality first, and pray. Most cancer survivors use all three.

As we learn about one part, we create changes in the others. That's why you can start wherever you chose: paying special attention to your body, mind, or spirit. Or, you may choose to begin by attending to two parts, or perhaps all three at once. The key is to find a healthy balance so that eventually, you are taking care of all three aspects of yourself. There is no special order, just your own intuitive order to find.

Using this workbook will help you find your own balance among mind, body, and spirit. You'll discover that as you take care of one aspect, all three change. How your body feels effects your mind. The state of your mind affects how your body feels. Practicing your spirituality eases your body and your mind. The state of your mind enables you to seek more spiritual...well, you see how it goes. It's all connected.

Listen to the CD, *Fighting Cancer,* first. With ease and comfort, it nourishes all three aspects at once. Then, choose what you want to learn more about, and begin. *I'll show you how.*

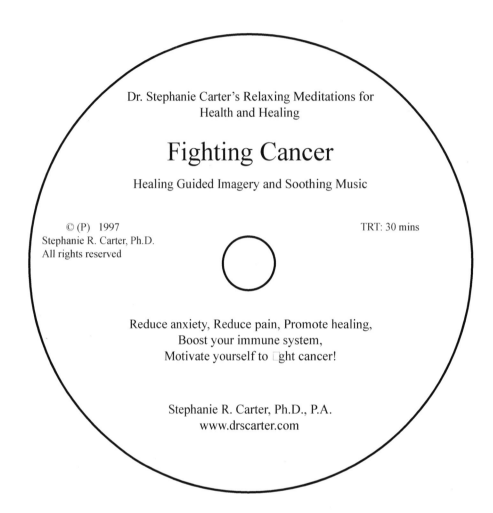

Dr. Stephanie Carter's Relaxing Meditations for
Health and Healing

Fighting Cancer

Healing Guided Imagery and Soothing Music

© (P)   1997
Stephanie R. Carter, Ph.D.
All rights reserved

TRT: 30 mins

Reduce anxiety, Reduce pain, Promote healing,
Boost your immune system,
Motivate yourself to ght cancer!

Stephanie R. Carter, Ph.D., P.A.
www.drscarter.com

Order your CD now.
Here's how:
Go to www.drscarter.com to order a CD or to download *Fighting Cancer*.
Fighting Cancer is also available on Itunes.

CHAPTER 1

Taking Charge

You First!
Fighting Cancer, Listening to the CD,
Boosting Your Immune System

*"In the midst of winter, I finally learned that there was in
me an invincible summer" (Albert Camus).*

First, put *yourself* first. *You* are now your first priority. This may be a new concept for you because you may be used to taking care of the needs of others before your own. Well, it's time to change that. You are starting the necessary journey to save your life, and to do that, you need to focus your attention on YOU. That's right. You come first. You must take care of yourself. That is your necessary and fundamental journey: learning how to take the best possible care of yourself in an organized, effective, and compassionate way. There are lots of things for you to learn about and explore, and in order to do those, you must make yourself the top priority. You can and you will.

This workbook teaches you how. You'll learn how to take care of your mind, body, and spirit. They are interconnected, and as you take care of one, you'll be taking care of the others. For example, as you learn how to relax your mind listening to *Fighting Cancer*, your body will relax, your immune system will be more powerful, and you will sleep better and reduce your pain. You'll reduce anxiety, clear your mind, and motivate yourself for the work ahead. You will be better organized and more involved with your medical treatment, and you will become more aware of complementary remedies, treatments, and activities that might help. You'll find that you may experience spiritual growth as you use inner resources you didn't know you have. All of this can happen as you simply play the CD, *Fighting Cancer*, listen, and relax. Please go to drscarter.com now and order the CD. Or, you can download it from Itunes or elsewhere on the Internet.

Embracing life

"It's never too late to start the fight for recovery. There are two reasons for that statement. The first is that whatever the stage of the illness when you start, you will probably improve the quality of your life. The second reason is that no matter when you start, there is the possibility that your actions may have a positive effect on the course of the illness. [Many personal stories illustrate] the power of the immune system…to kill cancer cells…it is reasonable for you to hope that your immune system can be bolstered to reverse the course of the illness. No matter what stage of the illness, every story of a recovered cancer patient teaches that same lesson" (Harold H. Benjamin, The Wellness Community Guide to Fighting for Recovery from Cancer, pages 7-8).

"Natural forces within us are the true healers of disease" (Hippocrates).

The first way you are going to take charge is by teaching your mind to calm your body. You're going to learn how to soothe your worried thoughts, let go of your fear, motivate and energize yourself. You will learn how to achieve success in your mind's eye. As you learn, you will reduce anxiety and pain, diminish side effects from treatments, and focus on being well. Your focus will move away from fearing death and illness, and move toward embracing life. To do all these things is really very simple. It all happens in the comfort of a favorite chair, within the quiet of a familiar room, as you listen to the CD. Let me explain.

About the *Fighting Cancer* CD

Fighting Cancer is a healing visual imagery relaxation exercise set to soothing music. It is designed to guide you through a mental rehearsal for a successful outcome in your necessary journey. As you listen, you will discover your inner motivation to move forward with the many demands of cancer recovery.

What does all this mean? How does it help? Let me review the terms.

Healing visual imagery creates a mind-body-spirit connection. It is the powerful use of your imagination as you use all of your senses. I think of it as a bridge that connects all the different parts of you: your body, your mind, your spirit.

All my life's a circle, sunrise and sundown
The moon rolls through the nighttime
Till the daybreak comes around
(Harry Chapin, Circle)

Using visual imagery is an ancient and effective form of healing. It's easy to do. It costs you nothing and requires only a small amount of your time. You simply allow pictures and images to form in your mind's eye. Imagine smelling aromas and fragrances. Imagine the sounds of things, the textures of whatever is around you, the temperature, and tastes. You simply allow yourself to discover your personal experience through whatever you are imagining. Images can be real or fanciful, from your actual experience, or from the deepest recesses of your own unique imagination. They can have conscious and unconscious meanings. You may understand the reasons why you chose certain images, or you may not have a clue why your mind chose an image. It doesn't matter what or why you choose, as long as your images are pleasant and feel good to you. Images just bubble up into your awareness and there they are.

*   *   *   *

Close you eyes for a moment and allow an image that is wise, strong, and comforting to bubble up into your mind. It might be a wise old woman or man, a ball of glowing white light, an animal, or anything else. One young man imagined a baseball field. He felt peaceful and energized, and his body felt cool. Write down any images that come to your mind and refer to the Feelings Chart in Chapter II to record what the feelings and accompanying sensations are for you.

_____

_____

_____

_____

_____

_____

By mobilizing the power of your mind you can improve your body chemistry. It changes the way you feel. Using imagery can affect your breathing, heart rate, blood flow, blood pressure, immune function, temperature, waking/sleeping rhythms, digestion, and sexual function. What a powerful mind you have.

I know that you are good at using imagery already because I know you worry about cancer. Every time you worry, you are imagining something negative, and you feel the matching sensations in your body. (Review the FEELINGS CHART in Chapter II if you need help identifying your matching body sensations.) When you worry or picture something negative, you may sweat, speed up your heart rate, or get a stomach ache. Your adrenaline and cortisol levels might surge, setting off a cascade of stress related biochemical changes in your body. See how powerful your mind is? And what about when you picture sad things in your mind? Your body reacts as if the sad event were actually happening. Well, just as you use your mind to feel worse, you can use that same power to feel better. Imagining positive and healing images will cause your body to respond, "Okay, this is what must be happening," and it will produce healthy physical reactions, and you will feel better.

"The bodymind responds to vivid images "as if" events being imagined were actually happening in the outside world. If you imagine you are running, your nerves and muscles produce slight but perceptible movements that can be detected with an instrument called an electromygraph (EMG). When you imagine hearing or seeing an object, the part of the brain – the auditory or visual cortex- registers it as though you had perceived it in the physical world...Imagery results in sparks of electricity and showers of chemicals permeating your whole being...Several studies have measured the output of the salivary glands when subjects are asked to think of a lemon. Try this yourself to test the connection between your image and your cells. You will note that the more senses you involve in your imagery – the color and sound of the juicy lemon, the felt sense of swallowing, the pungent taste – the more response you will feel" (Jeanne Achterberg, Barbara Dossey, Leslie Kolkmeier, Rituals of Healing).

Relaxation exercises have been studied for many years. Researchers find that people who practice various forms of relaxation exercises feel calmer, experience less anxiety, feel less pain, sleep more soundly, and report feeling generally better. Heart rate and respiration rate slow down, muscle tension relaxes, and blood pressure goes down. My patients who use relaxation exercises consistently report that their moods improve, they feel more optimistic, and they experience a greater sense of well-being.

Dr. Herbert Benson of Harvard Medical School outlines four elements necessary to achieve what he calls the "relaxation response."
1. **A mental device.** There needs to be a constant stimulus of some sort to shift the mind from logical, externally oriented thoughts.
2. **A passive attitude.** When distracting thoughts intrude, and they will, simply let them go as effortlessly as they came and redirect your attention to your focus, such as the *Fighting Cancer* CD.
3. **Decreased muscle tension.** You should be in a comfortable position so that minimal muscle work is needed.
4. **A quiet environment.** Choose a quiet place with as few distractions as possible. Often, it helps just to get comfortable and close your eyes wherever you are.

"Finding sacred places in your own house where you can sit and think, play tapes, CD's, etc. is important. You can really do this in your own home. Meditation is a place of freedom inside" (Ofelia, daughter of cancer survivor).

Soothing music helps you relax. One of my patients said to me, "Well, that's a no-brainer!" and we laughed. Of course, you know this too. You know the changes that happen in your mind, body, and spirit when you listen to music you enjoy. Music can be experienced in an emotional way, on a deeper level that feels very different from your conscious mind. In his book *Meaning and Medicine*, Dr. Larry Dossey talks about the musical melodies found within our DNA. Music is processed in your brain differently from language. Our bodies reflect sounds we hear right down to the biochemical level. It is an activity experienced by your body with more direct pathways to the most primitive parts of your brain. It represents associations, meanings, and symbolism from your past and present, as well as your hopes for the future.

You know how certain music transports you immediately to a different time and place? Music can perform that same magic for you now. Take advantage of this powerful tool.

"Music is the shorthand of emotion. Emotions which let themselves be described in words with such difficulty are directly conveyed…in music, and in that is its power and significance" (Leo Tolstoy).

On *Fighting Cancer*, you'll hear a soothing arrangement of Pachelbel's Canon in D, arranged in a way that will help you become quiet and calm. It was composed in the 17th century and is a peaceful, positive, and repetitive composition, ideal for calming you and focusing you on mobilizing your immune system to fight cancer.

$$* \quad * \quad * \quad *$$

Here is some of my favorite relaxing and motivating music:

- *Beethoven's 9th Symphony*
- *Mozart's Eine Kleine Nachtmusik*
- *Barbara Streisand's Higher Ground*
- *Righteous Brother's Unchained Medody*
- *Harry Chapin's Circle*
- *Willie Nelson's or Bette Midler's Wind Beneath My Wings*
- *Write your favorite relaxing and motivating music:*

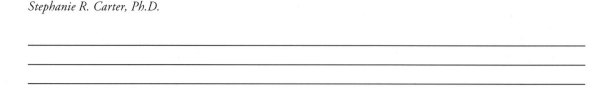

Mental rehearsal means that *Fighting Cancer* is designed to help you practice positive thinking skills and imagine healthy behaviors that will help you achieve a successful outcome.

Getting the Most Out of Your CD, *Fighting Cancer*

I created *Fighting Cancer* to help you reduce anxiety, reduce pain, calm your feelings, promote healing, and boost your immune system. This is all designed to motivate you to work hard and take charge of your fight against cancer, and to help you recover. It helps you feel more in control of yourself during this difficult time. It's calming, soothing, and motivating. It will energize you to fight, to keep moving toward your recovery. It is designed to restore and reinforce your positive thinking. It may even help you deepen your spiritual beliefs.

If you haven't already, it's time to listen to *Fighting Cancer*. Take it out now, find a comfortable, relaxing place to be, and simply listen. I will guide you through the whole experience. Everyone's experience is different. Just notice what *your* experience is. I'm sure that your mind will wander at times. Everyone's mind is busy, especially at a time like this. As you notice stray thoughts wandering in, simply say "oh" to yourself, and let them drift out as effortlessly as they drifted in.

Most people listen to *Fighting Cancer* in the morning. They find it calms and motivates them and gets their minds positively set for the rest of the day. Many listen to it two or three times a day.

"I wake up in the morning and sometimes I'm in sheer panic and I can't bring myself to get out of bed. I put Fighting Cancer on softly and listen to it mindlessly without actually doing the visualization, I just listen. Sometimes I don't have the strength to participate in the visualization because I'm so distraught, that I just listen and let the CD take me into a relaxed state of mind, so that I feel the CD is working for me and it takes me to a more relaxed state of mind. Sometimes I listen to it over and over again. It relaxes me and I get rest, even when I haven't slept well. Whether I'm actively or passively participating I feel like the CD is still working for me and I'm just absorbing the knowledge from the CD unconsciously. I put myself in a relaxed state. It's calming and I can begin my day" *(Naomi, cancer survivor).*

You will listen to this CD many times, so you have plenty of time to take in everything you need from it. There is no need to rush, no pressure to remember what to do. Be as relaxed as you need to be, no more and no less. Whatever you do is fine. Your comfort and ability to participate and take charge of your healthcare will grow every time you listen. That's right. You're doing very well.

Listen to this CD as many times as you can. The more you listen, the more your body and mind will respond to the positive messages.

Okay. Now you've listened to *Fighting Cancer*. Let's talk about what you heard and how you can use your imagination, that wonderfully creative part of your mind, to enhance the effects of the CD.

What is Cancer?

Cancer is a group of diseases characterized by the growth and spread of abnormal cells. It helps to learn all you can about your specific diagnosis. Staging describes the extent or spread of the disease from the site of origin. This information is essential to you and your healthcare team in determining the choice of therapies. The stages are I, II, III, or IV. Stage I is the earliest stage, stage IV is advanced. Please know that even people with Stage IV diagnoses can and do recover. They also go through the necessary journey, working hard for victory, just like you.

Your Immune System

In *Fighting Cancer* I told you that your body experiences cancer cells as invaders. Your body knows that cancer cells do not belong to you. Your body has an incredibly effective way to destroy cancer. It's called your immune system. Researchers who study psychoneuroimmunology, the combined study of psychology, the immune system, and the nervous system, have found that a strong immune system can keep you healthier. Long term stress and negative emotions wear down your immune system. Pleasing and positive emotions build up your immune system. Relaxing your body enhances your immune system. Positive thoughts enhance your immune system.

Cancer cells are always in everyone's body. Your immune system is always busy killing cancer cells, viruses, and bacteria. What you are learning when you listen to *Fighting Cancer* is how to boost your immune system to kill cancer. This highly personal work happens along with all your medical and complementary treatments. It is in addition to, not instead of, your medical and other treatments.

Your immune system is your system of self, with the remarkable ability to tell the difference between yourself from your non-self. It can tell friend from foe. It can tell the difference between your healthy tissues and cancer. It recognizes and destroys cancer cells, while defending your own tissues. It can do this because the cells in your own tissues and organs carry your unique identity card, lodged in the outer surface of your cells. They stand as strong flags of your identity.

*   *   *   *

You can create your own unique identity card by making your own personal identity flag. Draw a flag in whatever size you'll post some place where you'll see it often. Draw something in the flag that represents you and your good health. Use colors. Make it unique. People draw trees, landscapes, animals, themselves; whatever comes to mind and feels healthy and energizing is right for you.

Right now, your immune system cells are surveying your chemical markers on every single cell and molecule in your body, destroying invaders, and protecting friends. As your immune system detects cancer, it launches a well-organized, powerful attack, and kills the cancer. Scientific research has shown that people are able to enhance this activity by doing things like listening to *Fighting Cancer*.

Your immune system is a remarkably complex group of cells, known as white blood cells, which perform like an army of internal soldiers to guard against invaders. Your personal army can cleanse your lungs of foreign invaders, rid your bloodstream of infectious viruses and bacteria, and destroy cancer cells wherever they appear. They are your internal bodyguards.

Immune system cells attack invaders in various ways, such as surrounding and destroying, swelling up to become large and powerful, meshing together to move rapidly in a connected flank, encircling the enemy with long extended feet, injecting deadly chemical enzymes into invaders, and ingesting the enemy for later disposal out of the body. Your white blood cells stalk invaders, always on the prowl for what does not belong in your body. Forever alert and vigilant, they move into action to kill, digest, destroy, and remove anything unnecessary to your good health. All the while they are communicating with each other and with other cells in your body. Yes, this is what you have working for you deep inside your body. Like any other army, they are most effective when they have plenty of support and less distracting stress. *Fighting Cancer* provides you with more support and less stress.

Your immune system cells are your internal bodyguards. Some of their names are natural killer cells, T-cells, B-cells, neutrophils, and macrophages. These cells hunt, kill, and scavenge bacteria, viruses and cancer cells as well as the old dead cells of your body. They protect you day and night.

We also know that immune system cells can learn new behavior. In 1974, Robert Ader was giving immune-suppressant drugs to white rats. He gave them saccharin sweetened water followed by an injection of a drug to suppress their immune system. It did suppress their immune systems. Later, when he gave the rats the sweet water without the drug, their immune systems became suppressed again. He was startled to learn that immune system cells learn new behavior!

Other studies have shown that by relaxing deeply, you may be able to enhance how your immune system works. You may be able to further mobilize the help you need.

At the University of Massachusetts Medical Center, patients with diverse medical conditions including heart disease, diabetes, chronic back pain, colitis, and cancer learn mindfulness meditation to feel better.

At Ohio Sate University College of medicine, second year students undergoing the stress of final exams were taught a relaxation technique similar to *Fighting Cancer*. Blood tests of immune function showed that the stress of exams weakened the student's resistance to viruses. But the students who practiced the relaxation exercises most diligently showed the least impairment of resistance.

At hospitals all over the country, children with chronic pain from cancer are taught to escape it by visualizing themselves in a happy, relaxed place, and they report feeling better.

Using Immune System Imagery

In *Fighting Cancer*, I ask you to imagine your immune system at work fighting cancer. This is a very personal activity. Everybody does it in his or her own unique way. Some people imagine their immune system cells at work by picturing the actual cells in their mind's eye. They imagine the immune system cells killing cancer cells and then flushing the dead cells out of the body. Other people develop images that represent this process. For example, I imagine my immune system cells as large, powerful, polar bears that prowl around my body and swat invaders with their huge menacing paws. I imagine the invaders in various ways. Usually they are fish. In my imagination, I send the polar bears to the areas of my body needing special attention. They communicate with each other, find the fish that do not belong in my body, and eliminate them to protect me. I keep a few polar bear figurines in my office and in my home. They constantly remind me of the powerful bodyguards I have within myself.

You can imagine your own internal bodyguards at work either as they are in reality or as they spontaneously emerge in your imagination. It really does not matter. Your body does not know the difference. Either way works equally well.

Some people prefer very aggressive imagery, while other people are more comfortable with assertive, yet gentle imagery. Most of my patients begin imagining the cells as they actually are. After they have listened to *Fighting Cancer* a few times, however, their creative personal imagery starts to emerge.

*   *   *   *

Here are some examples of personal symbols which some of my patients have imagined.

- *Pacman face gobbling dots*
- *Sharks eating smaller fish*
- *Torpedoes destroying floating objects*
- *Ball of healing light cleansing areas of the body*
- *Laser beams of light burning their targets*
- *Healing colors moving through the body strengthening what is healthy and eradicating what is not healthy*

Write images that bubble up into your awareness:

_____
_____
_____
_____

Using Art

Many people find that drawing symbolic representations of their internal bodyguards is very helpful. It makes their imagery more vivid. This is an excellent way to further understand your feelings. You can do this, too.

*   *   *   *

First, get some really large paper. What is happening to you is a really big thing. You need space to express yourself. Get crayons, chalk, paints, colored markers, whatever color medium you like. Take in a few deep breaths and let yourself go. Use the whole paper, taking up the entire large sheet, even if you feel afraid at first. That's all right.

1. *Draw the cancer as you imagine it in your body.*
2. *Draw your immune system as you imagine it destroying or eliminating the cancer.*
3. *Draw yourself cancer free.*

Place the drawings in a place where you can easily see them when you want, with #3 on the top, #2 underneath, and #1 on the bottom. It is #'s 2 & 3 that will help you with your visualization process.

As you recover from the cancer, your visualizations may change. As that happens, draw more pictures. Your unconscious mind thinks in concrete, specific, visual images. Drawing them helps you visualize your personal symbols more clearly.

Creating Your Unique Relaxing Imagery

You can create hope and calm in any situation. There will be times when you don't have your CD with you and you need to relax. You can do the following exercise and take a vacation in your mind, and you can add your immune system imagery if you wish. Once you know how to do this exercise, you can do it anytime, anywhere, in just a few minutes. I often teach this exercise in my practice because it is good for whatever ails you.

*   *   *   *

CREATE YOUR OWN RELAXING IMAGERY

Close your eyes as if pulling down a shade to the outside world.

Take three deep breaths, saying to yourself: "I'm breathing in relaxation and breathing out my tension and worries."

Count down from three to one, knowing that you are relaxing more and more with each count down.

Imagine yourself in a comfortable and wonderful place that is pleasant, relaxing, and soothing for you. It might be a place that you have visited before, a place that you have seen in a magazine or movie, a place that you have heard about, or perhaps a place that exists only in your imagination. Wherever that place is, imagine yourself there. In your mind's eye, sit or lie down somewhere in this place, or perhaps you might feel more comfortable walking slowly on a path. The important point is that you feel comfortable, relaxed, and interested.

Imagine yourself experiencing all of your senses so that this place feels real to you. Remember that

11

if you focus your imagination, your body will respond as if you are really there. In your mind's eye, you are there, as you focus your attention on your:

- *SIGHT: see what is around you*

- *HEARING: hear the sounds of your place*

- *SMELL: smell the fragrances and aromas*

- *TOUCH: touch the things that are near you so you know what they feel like, feel the breeze on your skin, the temperature of the air*

- *TASTE: is there any taste in your mouth, such as salty sea air?*

- *AWARENESS: let yourself become aware of what you feel like here, let yourself relax and feel the comfort for a while*

When you are ready to end this exercise, count up from one to three to yourself, and as you do, reorient yourself back to your immediate surroundings, and open your eyes. Or, if you have time and you are in an appropriate place, you may wish to relax for a longer time, or drift off for a nap or to sleep for the night.

Just as any new skill improves with practice, doing this exercise many times will enhance your body's relaxation response. After you have practiced it many times, you will find that this exercise can be effective for you in just 2 - 3 minutes, anywhere, at anytime; but, do not use this exercise while driving.

Remember to involve all your senses. Then your body, mind, and spirit will react as if you are really there. Enjoy!

Find a photograph, painting, or another reminder of your chosen place. Display it at home or at work. You can even carry the reminder with you. Once your mind and body have been conditioned to relax when imagining this place, just the reminder of it will help you feel calmer.

You may want to let a place that is enjoyable, comfortable and safe bubble up into your mind now and write it down. Or, you may want to wait until after you have tried the exercise. You may find that you imagine different places as you practice this exercise. That's fine. Some people like to draw a picture of their unique place. When you realize which reminders you would like to have with you, write them down to help you remember later.

*   *   *   *

Your Unique Relaxing Place   *Your Reminder*

- *The beach*   *shell*

- *Meadow*   *photograph*

- *Mountain top*   *magazine picture*

- *By a babbling brook*   *smooth stone*

- *Your bedroom*   *object from your room*

- *Favorite hotel notepaper with logo on it*

_____

_____

_____

_____

CHAPTER 2

Taking Charge

Understanding Your Feelings, The Translation Process

"I had entered another world, in which the ordinary events of my life had abruptly become irrelevant" (Musa Mayer, Examining Myself, pg. 23).

Understanding Your Feelings

The feelings you are experiencing now are normal. I know you're scared. You may be numb or terrified. You feel sadness along with your fear. You may feel that your body has betrayed you, that it's out of control. You're probably angry, maybe even furious that cancer has happened to you. You may feel guilty that you did something to cause cancer. You did not. Cancer happens to people who take great care of themselves as well as to people who do not. Whatever care you have taken of yourself, you did the best you could at the time.

Your sorrow may be very deep. You may be thinking about death. Some people die from cancer, and you may be afraid that will happen to you. At this point, I talk with my patients about their thoughts and feelings about death and dying, about telling people what they want them to know, and about getting their affairs in order. We begin to talk about religious and spiritual issues. If you feel the need to do that now, please take a moment to look through Chapter VI. It will help you develop and express beliefs that support and comfort you.

While cancer causes you to be keenly aware of your own mortality, at the same time it offers you the opportunity to fully realize just how precious life is.

I know you're experiencing grief, thinking about all the losses that happen with a diagnosis of cancer: the loss of your good health, the loss of your life as it was, the loss of a life not focused on cancer, loss of time at work, perhaps even the loss of your job, maybe even the loss of body parts, the loss of trust in a safe world, of family life being a certain predictable way, of feeling in control. All of these feelings and thoughts are normal. As you move on in your treatments and personal growth and development, having these disturbing thoughts and feelings will change.

Cancer is a big deal. It changes your life. You're going to learn here that it also has the potential to change your life in good and meaningful ways. I know you would trade learning these lessons for not having cancer, but that's no longer an option. Your only healthy option now is to do what you have to do, learn what you have to learn, and recover. Choose life. Choose wellness. You can do this with a positive attitude, plenty of support, and even with joy. You'll see. I'll teach you how.

Now, take in a long deep breath. Let it out slowly. Now do it again. That's right. I'm going to show you what to do to feel calmer, motivated, and prepared to fight for your life. Yours is a difficult battle, but you can win it. Did you know that the National Cancer Institute estimates that approximately 11.4 million Americans with a history of cancer were alive in January 2006? There are surely more today. That's a lot of good company for you.

"You can gain strength, courage and confidence by every experience in which you really stop to look fear in the face. You must do the thing which you think you cannot do" (Eleanor Roosevelt).

It's important to recognize your feelings so that you can identify them and use strategies to feel better. I'll teach you strategies that really work. At this time, you may be so stunned by the diagnosis of cancer that you are numb, or you may be experiencing so many feelings that you are confused or terrified. Take another deep breath and let it out slowly. Taking deep belly breaths is an excellent way to begin calming yourself and slow your rapid, anxious thoughts.

*   *   *   *

Find a comfortable place to sit. Put both hands on your belly so you can feel what is happening there. Breathe in slowly and deeply. If you are taking a deep enough breath, you'll feel your belly rise. Then slowly let your breath out. You can feel your belly get low and soft again. Repeat this breathing in and out for a few minutes. You will feel calmer, quieter, and refreshed. You know, whenever you are tense you breathe in a shallow way using only your upper chest. This tightens your muscles and sets off a whole series of stress responses. The antidote is so easy. Just change your breathing to deep belly breaths and you'll feel calmer as you change your biochemical stress responses.

No feeling is good or bad. Your emotions simply *are*. They are just sensations that give you information. Don't judge them. Don't judge yourself for having them. Don't evaluate them. Use them as information about yourself and what you need to do. They are an important source of information, and it's necessary to know what they are so you can do something about them. Here's a way to help you know your feelings.

"Courage is doing what you have to do when you're afraid. If you weren't afraid, you wouldn't need any courage" (Susie, A six year old patient).

The Translation Process

You don't experience your feelings in words. They are sensations. How do you feel right now? You may not know. You may know you have a sensation, but you may not know the name of it. To be able to choose words to express your feelings, you have to go through a translation process. The translation is helpful because once you label a sensation, it is easier to know what to do. Using the Feelings Chart in this chapter will help you develop a vocabulary to describe your feelings.

In the chart, you will find four different feelings states and words to express different intensities of each feeling state. By identifying each feeling and its intensity, you'll have access to invaluable information about yourself. You will know if you like the way you feel, or what needs to be changed. You can be in one, two, three, or four feelings states at the same time. When people are in more than one feeling state, as you probably are now, they often say they are confused. For example, when you were diagnosed with cancer, you might have felt numb. If you look in the chart, you'll find that means you were frightened. Feeling numb is one of the body's safeguarding responses. It helps to keep you from feeling overwhelmed, so you can do what needs to be done. At other times you may have felt terrified, furious, deeply sad, and even relieved at finally having an answer to what your symptoms have been about. Being in more than one feelings state is normal. It's so normal that there are many words that people use to describe more than one state. That's why you'll see some of the same words in different columns.

You also have body sensations that accompany your feelings states. For example, when Mary came in two days after being diagnosed with cancer she was in such shock that she couldn't verbalize how she felt. She had an upset stomach, felt jittery with a rapid heart beat, was having trouble listening and concentrating. She couldn't sleep well, and she worried a lot. After we worked together for a while, she realized that she was frightened, angry, and deeply sad about the diagnosis of cancer, and she felt relieved to find out that she could start right now to lessen her anxiety and feel better.

Mary learned that her body was the part of her that communicated her feelings first. She learned to pay attention to her body's sensations in order to learn her emotional feelings. This was a big revelation to her. Identifying her feelings and their accompanying body sensations, hearing that they were all normal feelings and reactions for a person just diagnosed with cancer, helped her feel better. She was relieved to know that she was about to learn how to calm her thoughts and feelings and get motivated for the necessary journey ahead. Of course, her physicians were monitoring her physical reactions, and by becoming more aware of her own body and mind feelings, she became a better reporter to her physicians .

FEELINGS CHART

This chart is important to help you translate your emotional and physical sensations into words so you can help yourself feel better and be a better reporter to your healthcare team about how you feel in mind, body, and spirit.

The Emotions

Happy	Sad	Angry	Worried
joyful	tearful	mad	afraid
relieved	blue	frustrated	anxious
cared for	sorrowful	furious	nervous
content	abandoned	irritated	scared
proud	hurt	aggravated	helpless
confident	ashamed	agitated	tense
excited	lonely	annoyed	timid
balanced	suicidal	explosive	petrified
terrific	broken hearted	fuming	trapped
peaceful	pessimistic	disgusted	paralyzed
successful	isolated	offended	embarrassed
satisfied	alone	outraged	apprehensive
good	disappointed	resentful	intimidated
okay	empty	wronged	frightened
calm	left out	impatient	cautious

Happy	Sad	Angry	Worried
relaxed	rejected	manipulated	insecure
grateful	remorseful	used	devalued
enthusiastic	neglected	seething	guilty
terrific	unloved	rebellious	shy
powerful	sorry	crazed	humiliated
in control	grief stricken	bothered	threatened
glad	bored	revengeful	numb

Physical Sensations
(Your Body Expressing Your Feelings)

If you are experiencing any of the following physical sensations, then it is important to think about what they mean. They could be alerting you to a physical change that you should report to your health care provider or they could be telling you that you are in one or more of the feelings states listed above. For example, if you have a stomach ache, you could have a virus, a reaction to a medication, or you could be anxious or excited about something. Or, if you are feeling energized, comfortable, and alert, then you know that what you are doing is agreeing with you, and that is also important information for both you and your health care providers. Check with yourself and learn your body's own personal language.

good energy	calmness	crying	muscle tension	rapid heart rate
tiredness	sleepiness	lethargy	pain anywhere in your body	
weepiness	cold	hot	exhaustion	comfort
discomfort	nausea	agitation	sweat	tremors
alertness	aches	illness	upset stomach	flexibility
stiffness	restlessness	bloat	focused	rapid breathing

There are other words that communicate distress, but are not specific to one kind of negative feeling. They are sort of like saying you have a cold. They say you don't feel well, but they do not say if you have a runny nose, a sore throat, a cough, or all of those symptoms. Some of those words are:

| depressed | stressed | unhappy | overwhelmed | uncomfortable |
| bothered | vulnerable | upset | distressed | disconnected |

Add some of your own words here:

_____

_____

_____

_____

_____

*   *   *   *

You may want to do a body scan. Sit quietly. Breathe in a few deep belly breaths and let them out, breathing in relaxation and healing, breathing out all your tension. That's right. Take a few moments now to focus on your breathing, noticing how it feels to breathe in, and how it feels to let that breath go. Now, let your mind become aware of any part of your body or mind that is tense, or hurts, or that simply comes into your awareness. Breathe into that special part of you, perhaps even imagining special healing light permeating the area. If you wish, scan your body systematically. Become aware of your feet. How do they feel? Imagine your healing light permeating through them. Then move up to your ankles, your shins, your knees…paying attention to how each part of you feels…all the way up to the top of your head. Then, allow your whole body to be bathed in the healing light. That's right. When you have finished this exercise, write what you have discovered about your body. That way, you will remember to give that part of your body or mind special healing attention by telling your doctor or other healthcare practitioner about it, or by taking care of it yourself. This exercise will help you become an expert on your own body and mind. It will help you become a better reporter to your healthcare team.

I recommend that you check the FEELINGS CHART throughout your necessary journey. If you find your feelings or physical sensations are negative, you will know that you have to focus on taking care of yourself in one or more of the ways you're learning about. If you are confused about how you feel, check the chart. You'll also be referring to it for help in logging how you feel so you can be a better reporter to your healthcare team about how you are feeling in body, mind, and spirit. Surviving cancer is a learning process, and your most important learning will be about yourself.

" One's own self is well hidden from oneself; of all mines of treasure, one's own is the last to be dug up" (Friedrich Nietzsche).

My patients often ask me if they are supposed to have positive thoughts and feelings all of the time. The answer is no.

"Give yourself permission to cry" (Mickey, cancer survivor).

Recovering from cancer is a difficult road. It's only natural that your mind will drift to negativity at times. But when it does, you are going to know what to do to bring yourself back to a positive, proactive, and motivated place. You can. You will. You already are. That's right.

CHAPTER 3

Taking Charge

Captain of the Team.
Integrative Cancer Care:
Medical, Complementary and Alternative Care

"Each patient carries his own doctor inside him. They come to us not knowing that truth. We are at our best when we give the doctor who resides within each patient a chance to go to work" (Dr. Albert Schweitzer).

"Healing is an art and a science. It is said that the soul heals and that science cures" (Myrna Brind).

Integrative Cancer Care

Integrative cancer care means using the best of conventional medicine along with complementary and alternative treatments and activities. One does not substitute for the other. They are used in combination. To create the best possible combination for you means that you'll make choices and communicate with your healthcare team so that they all know the different treatments you are receiving and activities you are doing. In this way, you will create an individualized, effective plan that is holistic and healing, using the best from holistic remedies and the best of modern medicine.

You Are the Captain of Your Healthcare Team

Your physicians and other healthcare workers are your PARTNERS in your recovery. However, *you* are the CAPTAIN and must take charge and become an active participant on your health care team. You can and must do this. Studies show that patients who take an active role in their cancer treatment can have better outcomes and a better quality of life. In my practice, my patients experience a deep growth and satisfaction because they take charge of themselves, participate with their healthcare providers, and persevere through a very difficult time. You can too. You have already begun.

You are an important member of your healthcare team. It is *essential* that you think this because what you think influences how you feel and what you do. Your body, mind, and spirit listen to what you tell yourself.

*   *   *   *

Take a moment and stand up. Okay, now sit down. How did you do that? How did you mobilize billions of cells to act in perfect harmony and stand up? You simply said to do it so deeply inside that you didn't even hear yourself say, "Stand up." That's the power of your mind, the power of your thoughts. You tell yourself what to do all the time, and then you do it.

I want you to say to yourself **"I can do this,"** and then say **"I am an important member of my healthcare team"**.

*   *   *   *

Take a moment now to inhale a breath, breathing deeply into your belly, and then let your breath out slowly. Put your hands on your belly and feel it expanding as you breathe in and feel it receding as you breathe out. That's right.

Say these two statements on your out breaths.

Breathe in. Breathe out saying ***"I can do this."***
Breathe in. Breathe out saying ***"I am an important member of my healthcare team."***
Breathe in. Breathe out saying ***"I can do this."***
Breathe in. Breathe out saying ***"I am an important member of my healthcare team."***
Breathe in. Breathe out saying ***"I can do this."***
Breathe in. Breathe out saying ***"I am an important member of my healthcare team."***

These positive statements are called **affirmations**. You'll be learning more about affirmations as you do the exercises in this workbook. Affirmations are positive statements you say over and over to affirm yourself. Repeating affirmations are one way to teach yourself how to consistently think positively. Think of affirmations as creating useful new circuits in your brain. Say them even if you don't believe them yet. Your mind will get used to hearing them, and your body will respond with, "Oh, this is what we think." Affirmations work, if you find the ones you need and then practice them.

*   *   *   *

*While you are repeating your affirmations to yourself, think of matching visual images. For example, when you say **"I can do this,"** you can picture yourself with two thumbs up. When you say **"I am an important member of my healthcare team,"** you might picture yourself sitting at a conference table with your healthcare team.*

Many of my patients write affirmations and put them where they can see them. Some write them on little cards and leave them in their wallets with their credit cards so they see them often. Some leave messages for themselves on their personal voice mail. Some write with dry erase markers on their mirrors so they see them many times a day. Think of where you can place your affirmations so that you see them often as your mind gets used to these positive, healthy thoughts. See Chapter 4 if you want to create your own affirmations now.

*   *   *   *

Places I can put my affirmations so I see them several times a day:

- *Stickies on the dashboard of my car*
- *Notes on my bedside table*
- *On my refrigerator*
- *With my credit cards*
- *Personal voice mail so I hear them when I call in for messages*
- *With dry erase markers on my bathroom mirror (try a little mark first)*
- *Make rubber stamps of your most important affirmations and stamp them on your daily to-do lists, or include them in your grocery list*

<u>*Your ideas:*</u>

_____
_____
_____
_____
_____
_____
_____
_____

You are already an active part of your healthcare team because you take charge of your mind and use your mind to calm your body. You're already learning how to soothe your worried thoughts, let go of fear, motivate and energize yourself. You have learned how to practice for success in your mind's eye. You can see yourself cancer-free. You are reducing anxiety and pain, diminishing side effects from treatments, and focusing on your well-being. Your focus moves away from dying and embraces life. You are listening to *Fighting Cancer*.

According to the National Cancer Institute (NCI), cancer is no longer the dreaded disease it was years ago. There are important improvements in detection and treatment as a result of the research funded since the passage of the National Cancer Act in 1971 that have resulted in lengthening survival. According to the NCI estimates, *the majority of cancer patients will be cured or will live longer periods of time following their diagnosis.*

Medical options for cancer treatments change frequently, as we learn more about the mind, body, and spirit. As you plan for your medical, complementary, and alternative care, you will learn all sorts of new information. Everyone is overwhelmed at first by the sheer volume of information, not all of it precise and some of it contradictory. Take a deep breath. You can do this. Millions of people have done it before you, and more than a million people are doing it right now. You can too. You are not alone.

What follows are guides to the information you need to learn and some suggestions for keeping track of all this new and changing information. You will not be able to write in all the information now. The following pages are set up for you to use and fill in over time. You may want to create larger versions of the sample charts I have provided.

Communicating with Your Healthcare Team

Who Are Your Team Members?
Members of your healthcare team will change as your treatment progresses. Keep a record of everyone, including their names, addresses, phone numbers, fax numbers, and email addresses.

"Develop a relationship with the people in your doctor's office. I bake stuff and bring it in" (Ofelia, daughter of cancer survivor).

Name	Address	Telephone	Fax	Email
Me:				
Family doctor:				
Office Manager:				
Family doctor's nurse:				
Oncologists:				
Office manager:				
Oncologist's nurse:				
Appointment secretary:				
Physician's assistant:				
2nd opinion oncologist:				
Surgeon:				
Radiation oncologist:				
Pain specialist:				
Chemotherapy nurse:				
Other Nurses:				
Psychologist:				
Pharmacist:				
Nutritionist:				
Exercise instructor/personal trainer:				
CAM Care practitioners:				
Cancer support group:				
Family:				
Friends:				
Clergy:				
Neighbors:				
Work associates:				
Health food store:				
Hospital:				
Ambulance:				
Others:				

There are No Dumb Questions

"Nothing is ever silly" (Jackie, cancer survivor).

Ask questions. Ask whatever you do not know but want to know. Many of my patients say they feel embarrassed about asking so many questions. Don't be embarrassed. This is your life. It is really okay to ask questions. Most doctors welcome patients with lists. In fact, many doctors like it when they see you so involved in your care. With greater involvement and understanding, you are more likely to comply with your treatment regimen and be a good patient and a good reporter about your health and side effects. By communicating with your doctors so clearly, they can do a better job for you.

Occasionally, you might meet with a doctor who does not want to take time to communicate with you. If that happens to you, look him or her in the eyes and say calmly and assertively, "This is really important to me. I need some answers in order to understand my options. I appreciate your giving me this time."

*   *   *   *

Write your assertive statement in your own words.

_____

_____

_____

_____

_____

Copy your statement onto the top of your list of questions so it's in front of you when you speak to your doctor. Practice saying your statement. Look yourself in the eyes in the mirror and rehearse it, or say it to a family member or friend. If you are anxious about being assertive, it's important that you practice. Rehearse for success, just as you're doing when you use the CD. You'll feel good about yourself and your doctor will answer your questions.

Sometimes my patients tell me that they have met physicians who, although they possess a great deal of clinical knowledge, still seem to have difficulty viewing medical care as a partnership between doctor and patient. If any of your doctors have this view, just accept that they are doing their best and ask your questions anyway. This is not the time to be too polite or fearful of offending anyone. Be diplomatic, of course, but ask what you need to know and be persistent. It really is okay for you to do that. If you find that your doctor cannot communicate with you, you do have the option to find another doctor.

"Since 2000 I've had breast cancer four times. I didn't get any information until now and now I'm thirsty for information. I'm going to deal with this. Now I'm going to fight. The minute you get diagnosed, get information. Your doctor and others can tell you about

groups, tapes, etc. Your mind needs to be prepared for whatever happens. You have to learn to look at the positive of every negative" (Mercy, cancer survivor).

There may be a lot to remember and you may feel overwhelmed by all the information. Cancer is a subject that may be new to you. You'll be anxious, and you may hear many new words and instructions. Write everything down. Take pen and paper and family members or friends with you. Do not rely on your memory even if your memory is good. The anxiety and fear you are likely to experience early in the process may interfere with your ability to pay attention and remember. The people with you can be your extra ears for listening and your extra hands for writing things down. Some people even take tape recorders so they can listen again later.

Prepare for your appointments. Write your list of questions before you get to the office and share them with whomever accompanies you. Talking about the cancer may produce anxiety and you may forget to ask some important questions, or you may miss some answers. Anxiety is distracting. It's normal in situations like this. Plan for it.

I have listed questions that my patients often ask their doctors. Look through them carefully and add your own. Copy the ones you need to take to different healthcare professionals.

<u>Questions</u>
What is my exact diagnosis?
What stage am I in?
Can this kind of cancer spread?
Exactly what does that mean?
Has the cancer spread? If yes, to where and how do you know?
Are you a specialist in this kind of cancer?
What tests have you used?
What is my prognosis?
Will I need any other tests right now? If yes, what are they?
What is that test like?
Will I need more tests later?
What are the treatment options?
Have you used them before?
Do I need surgery? If yes, when?
What are the surgical options?
Can you recommend a good surgeon with whom you have worked before?

I'd like to get a second opinion (or a third opinion). Do you have any recommendations?

Is there a medical center somewhere that specializes in this kind of cancer?

Will I need chemotherapy? If yes, what kind, for how long, and what are the side effects I can expect?

How do I find out about the different kinds of chemotherapy for this cancer?

Will I need radiation? If yes, what kind, for how long, and what are the side effects I can expect?

How do I find out about the different kinds of radiation for this cancer?

What symptoms should I expect?

What do I do if I have trouble sleeping?

What do I do if I have trouble eating?

How can I take care of myself during chemotherapy to avoid infection? What can I do? What should I not do?

What do I need to know about fever and infection? What are the symptoms?

Do you have other patients with this diagnosis who would be willing to talk with me?

Tell me about side effects and how you recommend I lessen them.

Nausea

Hair loss

Pain

Infection

Fatigue

Other side effects:

What do you do for pain management? I want to do whatever I can to lessen pain, and I want to plan for it now.

Do you know a doctor who specializes in cancer pain management?

How do I find out about clinical trials? Are there any in your office or in this geographical area?

Do you have any literature I can take home and read?

Nutrition – what is good for me now?

Hydration – is it important to drink water?

Is what I'm experiencing cancer, or is it something else?

Are you available to answer phone calls?

Who in your office should I ask for when I have questions in between appointments?

Whom shall I talk to find out what my insurance will cover?

How do I find out about other sources of financial help for cancer treatment?

Do you know about support groups and other psychological services?

Other questions:

_____

_____

_____

_____

Questions I have thought about in between appointments.

_____

_____

_____

_____

Remember, You Are the Team Captain.

Keeping Track

It is important for you to keep track of what is happening to you in mind, body, and spirit. That way, you'll learn how to take better care of yourself. You'll know what helps and what doesn't help. You'll also be able to tell your healthcare team what is happening and they will be better able to help you.

Many people keep journals. I am going to suggest a format for you, but please feel free to change it in ways that will be more convenient for you. Log your physical symptoms such as pain, fever, and side effects as well as your emotional feelings such as worry, fear, or depression. Ask your doctor about tracking symptoms, such as body temperature, chills, sweating, sore throat, cough, problems urinating, diarrhea, swelling, redness. Ask if your doctor wants you to keep track of your Complete Blood Count (CBC). You can include all this information in your *Personal Mind, Body, Spirit Log.*

Remember also to log when you feel good, such as a pain free morning, a good laugh, or a comfortable evening, and how you achieved that 0 – 3 rating. You can use the Feelings Chart in Chapter 2. By keeping a log like this, you'll be able to look back and see what you did that worked so that you can repeat what feels good. If you wish, make copies of the following log and keep them in a file or a loose leaf notebook.

Personal Mind, Body, Spirit Log

Rating Scale for How I Feel Today

0	1	2	3	4	5	6	7	8	9	10
None		a little			medium			a lot		severe

Date/time	symptom/ feeling	# rating/ 0 – 10	what I did for relief	did I get relief?	Do I need to do anything further?

Calendar

Take charge of making your appointments and communicating about them to your different healthcare team members. You are in charge of preparing for them and following through afterward according to the instructions given.

Keep a calendar of appointments. It will help you stay organized and see where you have been, where you are now, and where you are going. It should include space for appointments, questions to ask, what needs to be done to prepare for the appointment, and what action steps will follow the appointment.

Information About Treatment Options.

As you learn more about your diagnosis, as you get second and maybe even third opinions, as you talk to people who have survived the kind of cancer you have, you will likely learn that you have treatment options. Get a separate notebook for recording what you are learning so that you can easily review the information as you make your choices of healthcare providers and treatments. Your page may be set up something like this:

Date: _____

Doctor: _____

Contact information: _____

Treatment: _____

Advantages: _____

Disadvantages :_____

Keep Your Own Copies of Your Medical Charts.

Many cancer patients keep copies of the information from their medical charts. At times, this may include x-rays, cell scans, CBC records, medications, etc. Speak to your doctor about this. If you have several doctors, which often happens, both you and they might appreciate your having this information to bring with you to appointments. Then, everyone will be clear about which treatments you are taking and your side effects, medications, and progress.

Pain

Although many people never experience pain during their cancer treatment, it is still important to learn about pain management right away. There are doctors who specialize in cancer pain management. Please ask your oncologist about who he or she recommends. *Call that pain specialist's office now* and ask when to get medical attention for pain for the type of cancer you have and the type of treatments that are planned for you.

*   *   *   *

You have already learned about communicating about pain in your Personal Log using a rating scale from 0 – 10. The following are some things you can do if you are in pain.

- *Write it down to discuss with your doctor*
- *Listen To Fighting Cancer*
- *Laugh*
- *Call friends and family*
- *Watch a movie that makes you smile*
- *Take pain meds*

Create your own list of what helps you feel better.

_____

_____

_____

_____

Managing Side Effects

Side effects mean that your treatments are working, but that does not mean that you have to suffer needlessly. Ask your oncologist and other healthcare providers what side effects you may expect and how to relieve them. Use your *Personal Mind, Body, Spirit Log* and tell them what is happening and ask what to do for relief. Remember that no question is too silly to ask. Many of the symptoms you may experience are temporary and there are ways to relieve them. If you don't ask, you may not know what to do and you'll worry needlessly.

Common Side Effects to Talk About With Your Healthcare Providers:
Below is a list of some side effects that you may want to discuss with your healthcare team. Fill in your own details and what you will do about them. Remember that it is comforting to be prepared, so write things down. Then, you'll have an easy-to–refer-to chart for you or your helper to read if the pain is difficult to manage.
Keep ongoing records in your *Personal Mind, Body, Spirit Log.*

*　　*　　*　　*

- Fatigue_____
- Pain_____
- Emotional distress (such as depression, anxiety, nightmares, frequent tearfulness)_____
- Infection _____
- Nausea_____
- Blood clotting problems (bruising, nosebleeds, headaches)_____
- Constipation_____
- Diarrhea_____
- Hair loss_____
- Problems with hands or feet_____
- Appetite changes_____
- Moth sores, throat and gum problems_____
- Tingling, burning, weakness, or numbness in hands or feet_____
_____
- Difficulty walking, balance problems_____
- Rectal soreness_____
- Skin problems_____
- Watery eyes_____
- Sexual concerns_____

Complementary and Alternative Care

Most of my patients use complementary and alternative care (CAM) in addition to their medical and psychological care. They do all the things you have been reading about in this workbook, and more. CAM care includes many different kinds of therapies that can offer comfort, healing, cures, pain relief, and solace. They are generally thought of as "mind-body" practices. They may include yoga, homeopathy, massage, therapeutic touch, flower essences, aromatherapy, reiki, acupuncture, naturopathy, Chinese medicine, and more. Although some are considered unconventional, in 1997, consumers spent an estimated $34 billion out-of-pocket for CAM care. Many physicians refer their patients to CAM care practitioners, and many of them offer CAM care specialists in their medical practices.

It is very important that you tell your physician if you are using any form of CAM care. Most patients who use CAM care never tell their physicians about it. Your doctor needs to know. This is really important. Some CAM care remedies may interact in powerful ways with medication you are taking, or some exercises or massage may be dangerous to fragile bones or to surgical recovery. Check with your doctor. Insist that your CAM care provider become a member of your healthcare team. Encourage them to communicate either with each other directly or through you.

There are No Dumb Questions for Your CAM Care Providers.

Ask questions. Ask whatever you want to know. Just as I encouraged you to ask your physicians and other team members anything you want to know, I also encourage you to ask your CAM care providers anything you want to know. You can ask some of the same questions from the previous list, and here are some others.

- What is acupuncture, massage therapy, homeopathy, or _____?
- Is there any scientific research about its effectiveness?
- What is the theory of how it works?
- What exactly happens during the treatment?
- How can it help me?
- How can I tell if it's helping me?
- Have you helped people with this kind of cancer before?

- May I speak with them?

- Is it safe?

- What are the side effects?

- What are your safeguards against spreading infection?

- Are you licensed or certified? By whom?

- What is your training?

- How does this treatment interact with the treatment I am receiving from my physicians?

- How much will this cost?

- Is it covered by my insurance?

Exercise

Exercise can help you feel better in body, mind, and spirit. Many of my patients tell me that they look forward to classes in Tai Chi, gentle yoga, walking, and even dancing. They smile when they tell me about it. If you are able to exercise, ask your doctor what restrictions you might have, and then try to find instructors who are knowledgeable about working with cancer patients. Be sure to choose an exercise that is appropriate for you: one that will help heal (not hurt) your body, soothe your mind, and comfort your spirit.

Nutrition

You know that you must take as good care of your body as you can. This includes nutrition. I suggest that you find an excellent nutritionist who can advise you about eating healthy foods that reduce inflammation and guide you about vitamins, supplements, and herbs. Like all the other aspects of cancer care, discovering the right food program for you will be an important part of your journey. My patients tell me that one of the many lessons they learned during their cancer treatment was proper nutrition. The changes they made during their treatment phase stay with them later.

Hydration

Drinking enough water is necessary. Please check with your healthcare providers and find out how much liquid you should drink every day. How much of it has to be water, how much can be other liquids. Ask.

You are taking very good care of yourself. You are being an effective captain of your healthcare team. What you're learning now will stay with you always.

CHAPTER 4

Taking Charge

Positive Thinking = Powerful Mind

You Gotta Have Hope
"Our life is what our thoughts make it" (Marcus Aurelius).

You are already moving forward on your necessary journey toward wellness. You are listening to the CD, you are learning how to calm your body and mind, and perhaps you've opened up your heart to a spiritual connection. You have become knowledgeable about the cancer diagnosis, what it means, and what to do about it. You are assembling a healthcare team you trust, and you can communicate your thoughts, feelings, and questions to them. You have even learned how to communicate with your own body and boost your immune system.

You can do so much already. Research has shown that cancer survivors have a fighting spirit and refuse to be helpless or hopeless. They change their lifestyles. They change how they handle stress. They are tuned into their own psychological needs, and they take care of themselves. They communicate about cancer. They see themselves as team members, taking responsibility for their health. This next section will give you more important tools for achieving those characteristics for yourself. Remember, by simply listening to *Fighting Cancer* you already have a good start.

Positive Thinking Makes a Powerful Mind

How you think affects how you feel and how you behave. How you perceive what is happening to you creates your experience. How you experience situations affects your mind which in turn affects your body.

Just think of a time when you saw something so beautiful that it moved you. Perhaps it was the ocean, or a panorama of gorgeous mountains, a glowing purple and pink sunset, or maybe your child's face. Think of the sounds, of the smells, how you felt then and how you feel now as you recall the sight. Can you feel the difference in your body? Your body is reacting to your thoughts. You are telling yourself, "That's beautiful," and your body is responding. That's what we mean when we say, "That moved me."

Situations do move us. When we perceive something as positive, our bodies respond with healthy good-for-us reactions. When we perceive something as threatening, our bodies respond with stress responses. Unfortunately, when stress responses continue for a long time, our bodies respond with unhealthy not-good-for us reactions. As you fight cancer, it is important to minimize stress and keep a positive attitude. There is nothing you can do about having been diagnosed with cancer. But there is a lot you can do about your perception of what is happening to you. There is a lot you can do to feel better now and set yourself up for the best chance of recovery.

Our perceptions are created by our internal self-talk. We talk to ourselves all the time. This inner self-talk is often so quick that we do not realize what we are thinking. I am sure that some of your inner self-talk went like this when you first heard the diagnosis of cancer. My patients often start out with some not-true negative thoughts such as:

- "This cancer will kill me."
- "I'll never find out what to do."
- "I won't be able to handle this."
- "Cancer treatment is too painful and too drastic for me."
- "There's nothing I can do about this."
- "My family and friends won't be able to handle this."
- "I feel guilty when I put myself first."
- "I'm scared and I know I will always be scared."
- "I'll never trust my body again."
- "I should not allow any negative thoughts to creep into my mind."
- "I should be able to handle this better."

Let's challenge each of those self-talk beliefs that create the feelings of fear and anxiety. By discovering why each statement is NOT true and then CHANGING your belief, you will change your experience of cancer recovery from one of fear and dread to challenge and growth.

"All things are possible until they are proved impossible – and even the impossible may only be so, as of now" (Pearl S. Buck).

I will start by challenging your thinking and offering suggestions for change. When I do this with my patients, I give them a sheet of paper to write down positive statements in their own words. If my words feel awkward to you, feel free to change them into whatever is comfortable for you. Then, I'll show you what to do with these powerful changes.

* * * *

Creating Positive Thinking for a Powerful Mind

"I know cancer will kill me." This is not true. Chances are high that you will not die from cancer. Millions of people have survived all sorts of cancers. You can too.
Positive thought: *Other people have survived this. I will too. My victory is inevitable.*

Your words:

_____
_____
_____
_____

"I'll never find out what to do." This is also not true. By reading this workbook, listening to *Fighting Cancer*, selecting and consulting with your healthcare team, talking with your support group, reading books, and finding information on the internet, you are already discovering what to do.
Positive thought: *I'm already finding out what to do. As I move on in my recovery, I will learn even more. I am capable of finding the best care.*

Your words:

_____
_____
_____
_____

"I won't be able to handle this." You *can* handle this. Think back about all the hardships in your life. You may not have known how to handle them at first, but somehow you learned, and you handled them. Now they are in the past. You will use those same skills here, and you are already learning new skills for handling serious problems. Sometime soon, this too shall be in the past.

Positive thought: *I can handle this. This too shall pass.*

Your words:

_____

_____

_____

_____

"Cancer treatment is too painful and too drastic for me." Not all cancer treatments are painful and drastic. Whatever cancer treatment you need, you will do. You will find out how to manage pain by seeing a pain specialist early in the process if you need one. You will find out how to manage side effects. In fact, you have already learned some pain and side effect management techniques by listening to the CD included in this book.

Positive thought: *I can handle cancer treatment. I learn skills to minimize any pain and side effects. I ask for what I need.*

Your words:

_____

_____

_____

_____

"There's nothing I can do about this." There is a lot you can do. You are already doing it. Although there may have been nothing you could do to prevent the cancer, there is a lot you can do to help yourself in body, mind, and spirit.

Positive thought: *I am doing many things to get well.*

Your words:

_____

_____

_____

_____

"My family and friends won't be able to handle this." Chances are great that your family and friends are stronger than you think. In another section, I'll talk about what to do and what to say to your family and friends. Yes, they will have their feelings of sadness, fear, and anger, too. That's normal. Let them have their reactions. The only person's reactions that you can control

are your own. You cannot control their reactions. Do the best you can to communicate with them, and then focus on yourself. Remember, in this situation, you come first.
Positive thought: *My family and friends do the best they can.*

Your words:

_____

_____

_____

_____

"I feel guilty when I put myself first." You may have a history as a caretaker, the person who takes care of the needs of others before taking care of your own. Some of my patients have done this for so long that they are not even aware of their own needs. Now is the time for change. Your life depends upon it. You have already begun taking good care of yourself, learning about your needs and acting upon them. You deserve to put yourself first. Let others do the best they can to take care of themselves. That can be their gift to you. Let them give it.
Positive thought: *I come first.*

Your words:

_____

_____

_____

_____

"I'm scared and I know I will always be scared." You have a choice. Your experience will be whatever you tell yourself. If you continue to say this to yourself, then chances are great that you will remain frightened. But if you tell your body that you are calm and handling yourself, your body will respond as if that is what is happening, and it will happen for you. By changing your self-talk and doing things that are reassuring like listening to *Fighting Cancer*, you can maintain a positive emotional attitude.
Positive thought: *I am calm. I am finding peace within myself.*

Your words:

_____

_____

_____

_____

"I'll never trust my body again." Many of my patients lose trust in their bodies when cancer is found. If this has happened to you, please know that it is a common response that *will* change. As you learn how to calm your body by listening to *Fighting Cancer* and doing other relaxing techniques, as you move through cancer treatment and take care of yourself in many ways, your trust in your body will return.

Positive thought: *I'm learning new things about my mind and body. I trust my mind and body.*

Your words:

_____

_____

_____

_____

"I should not allow any negative thoughts to creep into my mind." Negative thoughts will creep into your mind. They creep into everyone's mind. You are doing very well at learning how to use your mind in a powerful, positive way. When the negative thoughts creep in, use the techniques you are learning to let them go and replace them with what you want to think.

Positive thought: *I am in charge of what I think. If a negative thought drifts into my mind, I let it go and think a positive thought instead. I listen to Fighting Cancer. I use affirmations.*

Your words:

_____

_____

_____

_____

"I should be able to handle this better." My patients worry that maybe they should be handling cancer recovery better. This is old performance anxiety. Whatever you are doing, you are doing the best you can. If you could be doing any better, you would. You are learning and growing and doing just fine. Yes, there is a lot to do. Step by step, you are doing it. Be kind to yourself. You deserve the kindness and compassion you offer to others.

Positive thought: *"I am doing the best I can."*

Your words:

_____

_____

_____

_____

You may have other not-true negative thoughts. It is important to identify them so that you can challenge them. Are they really true? Write down any negative thoughts you have, even if for now you believe they are true. It may take you a while to think of why they are not true. It may help to discuss these with a friend, with your support group, or with a therapist.

Remember, you are in the process of changing a negative situation of fear and dread to a challenging one of growth and learning.

Negative thought:

_____

_____

Positive thought:

_____

_____

Negative thought:

_____

_____

Positive thought:

_____

_____

Negative thought:

_____

_____

Positive thought:

_____

_____

Negative thought:

_____

_____

Positive thought:

_____

_____

Affirmations
Affirm Yourself!

"Work on overcoming fear. I've been healthy all my life. When I was diagnosed I was terrified, out of my mind with fear. Friends came through. Affirmations made it possible for me to handle sleeping, eating, and treatments. Your mind is so powerful. Nothing had changed but my mind and attitude. I went to the computer and wrote down my own affirmations. Affirmations, breathing, and attitude have been so important to me. They give you hope and make you stronger. Ones that I use a lot are "I've overcome a lot. I'll overcome this. This too shall pass." (Viviane, cancer survivor).

You are learning how to change your negative thinking into positive thinking. You are developing a powerful mind. Powerful minds can do amazing things.

At this point, some of my patients wonder, "That sounds great, but some of the positive thoughts that I want to believe don't feel natural. Inside, I still tell myself the negative thoughts. How do I change that?"

I tell them that will change with practice. Learning positive thinking skills develops with practice, just like learning to play tennis or learning how to walk. Some of you learned positive thinking skills as a youngster, and they may come easily to you. Others are learning them for the first time and it may take more practice. Either way, you can learn to increase the power of your mind to work for you in positive and healing ways.

Imagine that when you were little you went outside to play. You found some stones and lined them up. You discovered that two stones plus two stones equaled four stones. You moved the stones around in different configurations and much to your delight, they always added up to four. Well, you went inside to your family and proudly announced your discovery. To your amazement, your family told you that 2+2 = 5. You knew that couldn't be right. With your own eyes and hands you knew that 2+2 = 4. But, in order to get along in your family, you adopted their thinking, 2+2 = 5. In the beginning, it felt strange, but over many years, 2+2 = 5 began to feel right. Over and over again you used 2+2 = 5, with out being conscious of using it. You made errors in math problems, but generally you did okay, so it was not a big problem. As you got older, math problems became more complicated, and you never knew why your answers were always a bit off. When it became important to you, you went for help. Your math tutor identified your problem. "You always write that 2+2 = 5. That's wrong. Let's challenge your thinking and look at the evidence. See, these two stones plus these two stones equals four stones. You can count for yourself and see that it's true." Well, you could see that it was true. 2+2 = 4. But, it didn't feel right. Although you could see your mistake in thinking and clearly see reality, it just didn't feel right. It felt awkward to say 2+2 = 4. So how do you change that awkwardness so that your belief and feelings match the truth? Just as you once practiced 2+2 = 5 so many times that it felt natural, you begin to practice 2+2 =4 over and over and over, and as you do, you visualize counting the stones. Over time, especially because now you know it is true, 2+2 =4 feels natural to you. It starts to feel comfortable and true because you are saying it repeatedly, reinforcing what you can see is true.

It's the same with your not-true beliefs about cancer and your ability to handle treatments, let go of fear, and focus on your recovery. For example, "This cancer will kill me" is a statement based on the false belief that cancer is always a death sentence. That is an old, not-true belief. There are so many treatments, new ones being developed all the time, and wonderful oncology treatment centers all over the world. There is a lot of help for you. Approximately 11.4 million Americans with a history of cancer are alive right now and the number is growing every day. That's a lot of people. You can be one of them. The old statement "cancer is a death sentence" is a 2+2 = 5 belief that is not based on the evidence. You may have heard it so many times, however, that it became lodged in your unconscious and felt right. Cancer is a serious disease, but usually not fatal.

*   *   *   *

Your new 2+2 = 4 is the positive thought:
Positive thought: *Other people have survived this. I will too. My victory is inevitable.*
Your words:

_____

_____

_____

_____

Look around you for the evidence. Talk to people who have recovered from cancer. Read articles and books written by survivors. The good news is out there waiting for you.

*   *   *   *

Affirmations work when you use the ones you need and practice them. You have already started your list. Look back at the positive thoughts that you wrote in this chapter and list the ones here that you want to practice. Remember that over time, the affirmations you need may change.

_____

_____

_____

_____

Here are some examples of how people practice:

- *Listen to Fighting Cancer. You will hear many affirmations.*
- *Deep breathing in a relaxed state, and on the out breath say your affirmation.*
- *Place it where you see it often (see examples in Chapter 3).*

"Continuous effort, not strength or intelligence, is the key to unlocking our potential" (Winston Churchill).

"I am the Greatest!" (Muhammad Ali).

As you practice your affirmations every day, even when you feel you don't need them, you'll be ready to use them during those difficult times when you need extra help from yourself. Then, your affirmations will feel natural, comfortable and intuitive, like old familiar supportive friends, like 2+2 = 4.

Benefit Finding

Benefit finding means gaining emotional growth from an experience, even when that experience is traumatic. People who find benefit from having cancer might say things like "cancer has helped me appreciate my life more," or "cancer has helped me see priorities more clearly," or "cancer has brought my family closer together," or "cancer has taught me patience." Research at the University of Miami has shown that people who find that cancer had made some positive contribution to their lives had an increase in optimism, had better ability to return to regular life, decreased anxiety, less thought intrusions about cancer and less social disruption. So even though I know you would trade any new learning for not having cancer, that's not your choice. Your choice is to practice what you are learning: work at relaxing and reducing anxiety and pain (Chapter 1), work at expressing your feelings (Chapter 2), at thinking positively (Chapter 3 & 4) and be grateful that you are learning important life lessons. And there are more ways to find benefits as you read the next three chapters.

CHAPTER 5

Taking Charge

Connection, Communication, and Support

**"It may look like we run this alone, but we can only do
it with a whole team of people behind us"
(Deena Kastor, August, 22, 2004, interview on NBC TV immediately
after winning Bronze medal in the Olympic Women's Marathon).**

Staying Connected

Connections are important. In other chapters I have talked about connecting to *yourself* in mind, body and spirit through using visual imagery, meditation, deep breathing, by becoming aware of your feelings and thoughts, by paying close attention to your body, by becoming the leader of your healthcare team, and by exploring your religious and spiritual beliefs. In this chapter, I talk about the importance of connections to other people.

Most of my patients know what I mean when I talk about feeling "connected". You know when you feel connected to the people in your life. It's an intuitive knowing. It feels *good*. It's the process that happens between two or more people when they feel they communicate truth about themselves and that that truth is heard. Sometimes it even happens without words.

*   *   *   *

Close your eyes. Take in a few deep breaths and relax. Now think about a person to whom you feel connected. This may be a person you know intimately, or maybe someone you've just met. It really doesn't matter, as long as you feel the connection as you imagine being with this person. Now, pay attention to your thoughts. Pay attention to how positive thoughts have emerged. Feel the calmness in your body. Feel that some energy greater than yourself is involved. Feel the energy that you know exists between you, connecting you. Stay with this pleasurable experience for a few minutes.

Connection to other people is important. It is what helps you to grow and move forward in your journey to wellness. Connections will help you feel calmer and less isolated. You'll be able to help others as they offer help to you. You'll learn more than you can imagine right now.

A cancer diagnosis can be disconnecting. Any negative emotions are disconnecting. If you check your FEELINGS CHART in Chapter 2, you can see that any time you experience any of the emotions in the sad, angry, or worried columns, you might feel disconnected and isolated. Remember, you can be in more than one column at a time, so you might feel sad and relieved, or anxious and loved at the same time. At those times, connecting may be difficult.

Sometimes connections are automatic, they just happen. Other times, they take work. As time goes on, you are learning more about moving into the column of positive emotions. Staying connected to other people helps you do this. Just being connected to another person creates a positive feeling. It can comfort you in your sadness, calm you out of your fear, and motivate you to leave helplessness behind.

"There is great power within each one of us. Be aware that we are special human beings and have powers and gifts that we should welcome. Find people who will help you to recognize and experience growth in this quality" (Mickey, cancer survivor).

Asking for Help and Using Social Support

"Healing is the effect of minds that join…" (28-III-2).

Don't even think about making this journey by yourself. Get over the "I can do it all by myself" syndrome. Ask for help. Use your social support system, and build a bigger one. At the end of the workbook, I have listed some resources to help you expand your support system.

Using a social support network is a sign of good emotional health. It is good for you to have people around to connect to and to lean on when you need it. It is also good for them. It's hard for one person to do all that you might need, so expand your network to include people with different kinds of help to offer. This is, by the way, healthy at any time in your life, not just now when you have cancer. Your list might include family members, friends, co-workers, clergy, support group members, a cancer patient telephone buddy, an internet support group, librarian, neighbor, etc.

List your social support network. The list will change and expand over time.

NAME   TELEPHONE NUMBER   EMAIL

_____

_____

_____

_____

_____

_____

Find a Support Group

It is important to find a support group. Characteristics of cancer survivors include both the ability to talk openly about cancer and their compassionate involvement with other people with cancer. A support group provides a safe environment for you to develop these characteristics.

There is research emphasizing that group support for cancer patients improves psychological wellbeing, reduces anxiety and depression, and improves quality of life, coping skills and mental adjustment. There have even been studies showing that some people with breast cancer live longer. Support groups can counteract the feelings of helplessness and social isolation that many cancer patients feel. These feelings are correlated with poorer health outcomes and poorer quality of life. *So join a support group now.* Get yourself connected. It's good for you.

Support groups can be large or small. Some of them are for patients with any type of cancer. Others are organized for people with a specific type of cancer. Find out what is available in your area. You can make telephone calls or explore the internet. You might ask a friend or family member to help you search. Maybe one of your children wants to help.

Using Psychological Services

"There are certain things that are common with cancer, like with chemotherapy – certain blood counts can get too low and you have to have treatments to get them back up. Well, sadness, sorrow and fear are common emotional reactions to cancer. But when they become too intense, there needs to be an intervention to help ameliorate that. Because just like low blood counts can complicate your recovery, depression can complicate it if left untreated. Depression can deplete the immune system, make it harder to follow through on treatments, and doesn't keep your emotional stamina up" (Peggy Rios, Ph.D. Program Director, The Cancer Support Community of Greater Miami, Miami, FL).

Stephanie R. Carter, Ph.D.

How to Know When You Need Individual Psychotherapy

You may need individual psychotherapy if:

- your feelings are intense
- you do not experience enough relief from them
- you are feeling so numb that you can't feel anything at all
- you are feeling so isolated and disconnected that you cannot re-establish your connections with people
- your worry about yourself, family, or friends is overwhelming
- you cannot get organized enough to take charge of your treatments
- you can't get by the fear
- you want to discuss your issues privately in a one-to-one setting
- you are not complying with treatment recommendations
- you can't turn your racing mind off
- you need help that you're not getting in other places
- you are having trouble coping
- you simply want to come.

Some of my cancer patients come in for two or three sessions and find the relief they need. Others come in for a year or more. Some come in for a few sessions, then I don't see them for awhile, and they return to therapy when they need it. They seem to do their work in "chunks", or when something happens and they feel the need to come in and process their thinking and feelings. Many come to work out their feelings with a therapist because they don't have to worry about my feelings. They might worry about the feelings of family or friends or even support group members, but they can say what they need to say and not worry about me. Sometimes people need the time to work out their feelings and thoughts privately before they move on to working them out with other people. Therapy is a safe place to do this.

Many people come to therapy to work on grief. Grief is a normal response to a cancer diagnosis. You may need individual help to recover from grief because you may have a lot of losses to face. If you find that you cannot respond well to offers of support and comfort, if you are irritable often, if your attention and concentration are shorter than before, if you feel stuck in hopelessness and emptiness, if you feel angry, guilty, and your self-esteem is suffering, then I recommend you get help.

Being diagnosed with a life-threatening illness is traumatic and some cancer patients develop Post Traumatic Stress Disorder (PTSD). Even family members can develop this disorder. If you think you or someone in your family might be suffering from PTSD, please get psychological help right away. It is treatable. Some of the symptoms include intense fear and helplessness that trigger a re-experiencing of the trauma, perhaps in nightmares, flashbacks, and intrusive thoughts; persistent avoidance of reminders of the trauma like, perhaps, not wanting to talk about cancer or avoiding some treatments or doctors' appointments; and persistent increased difficulty with sleep, a hypervigilance such as overreacting to too many normal body aches and pains, and irritability that just doesn't go away. If these symptoms last for more than one month and cause you significant distress or make it hard for you to function socially, at work, or in other areas of your life, then please get checked by a licensed therapist.

Using Psychiatric Services

You may want to discuss using psychotropic medications with your therapist. These are medications that can help relieve depression, lessen anxiety, or help stabilize your moods. Sometimes, the use of medication *along with* talk therapy is the fastest and most effective way to get relief. In some states, specially trained psychologists can prescribe medications. Otherwise, psychiatrists and other MDs can always prescribe medications. Remember to tell your healthcare team about your individual therapy and about any medication you might be taking.

The Power of Telling

Okay. We've talked about the importance of getting connected, joining a support group, and getting professional help. Talking to people helps in your recovery.

Talking to people may be difficult for you, but with practice, it'll get easier. As a result of your talking with others, you'll experience an emotional growth and level of connection that is deeper than before because the feelings you'll be talking about are deep, intense, honest, and profoundly personal. This is good for you.

Now, let's talk about talking to the people in your everyday life. There is no "easy" way to tell people you have cancer. Just take a deep breath and say it. "I have cancer." Give yourself permission to show feelings. It's okay. People will do their best to handle your expression of feelings and most will try to comfort you. They know it's difficult for you. Although there is nothing they can say to make the cancer go away, their effort to connect and comfort can help you feel better.

You have a choice about whom to tell and when to tell. With the people close to you, it's best to tell them as soon as possible. Cancer happens to your family and friends as well as to you. Give them the time to deal with what's happening. Give them the opportunity to help you.

Tell people how they can communicate with you. For example, if you are tired and not feeling well from treatments, or if you are focusing on your daily treatments and do not want to be disturbed, you might tell family and friends that they can write you notes, or leave you messages on your answering machine. Tell them you may not get back to them regularly. Some patients leave updated messages on their answering machines so they don't have to return too many calls.

Others write periodic updates, make copies, and mail or email them to family and friends. Patients who are comfortable using computers create websites and blogs with updated information. Some children do this for their parents. *It is up to you to decide how much contact you need and how to receive it.* Of course, your needs will change during the course of your treatment. Remember that you are putting yourself first, so put a little thought into what you need, and communicate this clearly to the people around you. *Do not* cut them out of your life. That's a disconnection and that's not good for you. *Do* be clear about the amount and kind of contact you need. Communicate what you want to your social network. It's really good for you to state your needs clearly. Let them support you. You need the connection and so do they.

Telling Your Spouse or Partner

Tell your spouse or partner as soon as possible. Tell them as you or your doctor suspect cancer. Tell them as you go through the diagnostic tests and ask them to support you.

Tell your spouse or partner what you know, and if you feel comfortable and if they want to, include them in your search for information. *Be specific about what you need. Be specific about what you want.*

Share how you feel, what you think, your fears, your hopes, your dreams.

They will react in their own way. They may become business-like and task oriented and not show any feelings. Or they may be overcome with fear. If the cancer diagnosis causes a disconnection between the two of you, consider going for couples therapy. Therapy is a safe place to vent feelings, reconnect, and plan.

Your spouse or partner will have emotional reactions similar to yours. Encourage him or her to get help, if needed. Right now, your focus must be on your taking care of yourself.

Common issues that couples talk about are: your dying, the unknown, work, possible loss of income, handling responsibilities for the household, responsibility for children and pets, relationship changes, sexual intimacy changes, decisions about your treatment, who to tell, coping skills for all the tasks ahead, religion, spirituality, legal preparations for your death, and reminders to appreciate each other daily. *It's important to talk about ALL these things.* You may even want to put these items in a list, add your own thoughts, and talk about them with your spouse or partner. You won't have answers for them all now, but to open the discussion is healing. It's connecting, and that's good for you. Just giving you and your spouse or partner the permission to talk about these issues with you is calming. Get professional help if these conversations become too difficult.

How to Tell Your Children

One of the hardest tasks cancer patients have is telling their children that they have cancer. Everyone wants to protect their children from sadness and fear. No one wants to tell their child that they have cancer. However, *it's very important to tell your children what is happening.* Kids know when something is wrong. If you don't tell them what is wrong, they will interpret the situation in their own way, and very often, they interpret wrong and they interpret worse. Share your feelings with your children. Keep their lives as routine as possible. Tell them they can still play and laugh, visit friends, and go to school. Give them that permission.

"Tell people to encourage their children to go out and be with people and live their lives or they'll feel like they have to stay and they'll feel guilty about not being home. Although at times, it's good to be home too. Say "It's okay to go out and have fun." Kids should find a place that is the same as before cancer, like a friend's house, school, or some special place – an actual physical place -where no one is hounding you, that is, be with people who were close friends before and concerned about how you are doing but don't feel the need to press the subject all the time. You want to feel normal, like you felt before treatment. You want to feel normal and that things are okay. Find friends to help you do this"
(Brennan, son of cancer survivor).

Before you talk to your children, become aware of your own thoughts, feelings, and beliefs about having cancer. Talk to someone else so you get practice in saying whatever your thoughts, feelings, and beliefs are. Then, if your children ask questions, and they probably will, you'll be a little better prepared to explain to them whatever they need to know.

Look at the situation as an opportunity to help your children grow. You and your children may wish this hadn't happened, but it has. Look at this as a time to learn new coping skills and to teach them to your children. I know you'd trade the new skills for no cancer in a nanosecond if you could, but you can't.

Think about the age and maturity of your children when planning what to say and how to say it; then be guided by their questions. I'll talk more about the different ages later in this chapter.

Find a calm time when you (and whomever you might want to assist you) can be alone with your child or children. It's important that all your children know the same information (age appropriately, of course) so they can feel free to talk with one another. Tell them that they can talk with each other, and with you. Tell them who else in your family and friends network knows so they have more people to talk to. Remember, this may be frightening and disconnecting for them too, so they need to know their network of connections.

Tell your children in the most direct, tactful, and appropriate way you can. Ask them what they have heard, and then LISTEN. Ask "What is it like for you to hear this?" Then, listen more. Some children have lots of questions, others have none. Some react with outbursts of emotions, others seem like they don't care. Whatever your child's reactions are, accept them. Children generally don't tolerate upsetting feelings for long. They will often distract themselves. Adults think this means they don't care, but it doesn't. It's just your child's way of not becoming overwhelmed by the information. If you are worried about how your child is dealing with the cancer, treatments, and the effects it is having on the family, please get professional help.

Tell your children about you and cancer. Be honest with them. Give them small amounts at a time of age-appropriate information. Here are some guidelines for talking with your children.

Tell children as soon after diagnosis as you can. Children know when something is wrong, and if you don't tell them the facts, their imaginations will create facts.

Practice your explanation beforehand.

Show your feelings.

Give your children small amounts of information at a time, according to their ages and levels of maturity.

Make it clear that a cancer diagnosis does not necessarily mean death.

Remember that you may have to repeat what you say many times. It's difficult information.

Say, "I don't know", if you don't know.

Explain what cancer is.

Ask them what they have heard about cancer so you can dispel any myths.

Explain and prepare them for your treatments. They will assume that the treatments are *bad* because they'll see the side affects. Tell them the treatments are making you better and the side effects mean that the treatments are working.

Tell them that you have doctors and other health caregivers who are helping you get better.

Assure them that they will be taken care of and that their needs will be met. If your caretaking of them has to be interrupted, tell them who will look after them. Be very specific about these plans. Children worry about what will happen to them.

Tell them that they did nothing to cause the cancer. It is not their fault. Neither the cancer nor the treatments are punishment.

Tell them that cancer is not contagious. Children are used to missing school or play so they won't "catch" an illness. Children often mistakenly assume cancer is contagious.

Keep routines around the house as much like before as possible, including their personal daily routines. Routine is comforting.

Keep discipline and house rules as much like before as possible. This is comforting for your whole family.

Tell them that your family and friends are here to support you and your children.

Tell them how they can help as part of your family team.

Leave them with feelings of hope and tell them that even though you and they are upset now, there will be better times ahead.

If you have to be away for a treatment, stay in touch the best you can to reassure them that your illness has nothing to do with how much you love them.

Be prepared to discuss death. At around age 7-10, children begin to understand the finality of death, although, like everything else, the age at which they understand is variable. Do not use terms such as "like sleeping" for any age child. Death and dying are not talked about much in our culture, so you might find it helpful to talk with someone about death and dying before you talk to your child. Children often know more than you think, and it always helps them to talk about their concerns.

Tell them you will always love them, wherever you are. Tell them that now.

If you have trouble talking about any of these issues with your child, ask a trusted family member or friend to talk with your child. If that is not an option for you, find a therapist to help you.

Parents want to know about kids' reactions to talking about cancer. Children worry about many things, just like people of any age worry. I've listed the most common worries below. Be patient and take it slow. Most conversations with kids are short, and they will happen during the most mundane moments, like while giving a bath, eating a sandwich, washing dishes, folding clothes, riding in the car, playing a quiet game on your bed. Take the lead from your children. Listen carefully. Show your children you're listening by telling them what you're hearing them say. Kids like that. They know you are connecting to them.

> *Tell your children that their reactions are normal.*
> *It's ok to cry and feel sad sometimes, and it's ok to smile, have*
> *fun and play and forget all about it sometimes.*
> *Take their expressions of feelings seriously.*

Here are some common concerns.

FEARS THAT WORRY CHILDREN
- Death of loved one
- Death of self
- Separation from loved ones
- Cancer is contagious
- The cancer was caused by something they did, said, thought, or felt
- Life as they know it will now change
- No one will take care of them
- The unknown
- Loss of family security
- Parents are often afraid, so they are too, even if they do not know why
- Increased worry and fear in general

ANGER
- At you for getting cancer
- At you for leaving them for treatments and hospitalizations

- That cancer and cancer treatments upset their lives
- At what may happen in the future

SADNESS
- Because you're sad
- Because there are many losses to deal with
- Because there are many changes in their daily lives, e.g. it may be harder to have friends visit
- Because of grief reactions in the family

ISOLATION/SEPARATION
- Feeling left out
- Feeling different
- You may be busier, preoccupied, and gone more from their daily routine

CURIOSITY
- Asking lots of detailed questions

DENIAL OR EFFORT TO CONTROL OVERWHELMING FEELINGS
- Refusal to talk about cancer
- Refusal to talk about changes in the family
- Refusal to express feelings

Very young children generally do not need a lot of information. They are more interested in what is going on at the moment and what is happening to them. It's still important to tell them the word "cancer" because they'll hear it in conversation, but they won't understand what it means. Most young kids know about being "sick" because they have been sick. Be concrete when you speak with them. For example, "I'm not feeling well today so I will not be able to make your lunch. Your grandmother will help". All kids, particularly the younger ones, fear separation. So if you have to be separated because of treatments, call, leave photographs around, leave them with known, trusted adults.

Older children usually want more information because they understand more about what illness means. They are often interested in hearing about good cells and bad cells, they want to know what treatments are like, and why they affect you. They often get angry because life has changed and you cannot do all the things you used to do. Tell them it's normal to feel this way. They should not feel guilty.

You can say things such as "the medicines I take kill the bad cells and help the good cells". "I may look different right now, but inside, I'm still the same mommy".

Teenagers often find it hard to cope with cancer in the family. They are at the age when their primary interests are out of the home, and they often get angry that cancer is tying them to their family just when they want to get away. This is a normal feeling and you should tell them that. They do not need to feel guilty. Give your teenagers frequent updates about what is happening medically. Give the information in "sound bites", keeping it brief. They'll ask for more information if they want it.

Keep the lines of communication open. Some children want a lot of information, some want very little. Some need a lot of reassurance, others need little. Check with them. Ask others, such as your spouse, a trusted friend, or teacher, to keep an eye on them for you, so you know how they're doing. Are you telling them what they need to know? Would they like to know more? Less? Be sure to tell your child who else they can talk to, for example, their other parent, an aunt or uncle, family friend, school counselor, therapist, or clergy. Sometimes kids will talk about their feelings more openly with someone else because they do not want to burden you with their sadness, fear, or anger. Be open to getting professional help if you see your child's behavior changing in negative ways.

You are the expert on your child. You know what's "normal" for him or her. If you see any changes in behavior that last longer than about two weeks, call a psychologist or other licensed therapist. Sometimes it only takes a brief phone call to get the information you need to help your child. Some changes to watch for are changes in sleeping, eating, mood, habits, clinging behaviors, irritability, tearfulness, school performance, general behavior patterns, increase in frequency of stomach aches and headaches, and more accidents than usual.

Most children want to talk to their friends about cancer in the family. Give them permission to talk about it. Some children may want to rehearse with you what to say to others. That's a good idea. Which friends do they want to tell? *Think about this first, then talk about it with your child.* If you have a problem with telling others and want to keep having cancer a secret, please speak with a professional. Keeping cancer a secret is disconnecting for you and your children. If you have young children, I recommend that you talk to their teachers. Teachers can often help in knowing how well your child is adapting to having cancer in the family. They can also be a wonderful source of support and connection for your child.

*   *   *   *

You're going to be teaching your child about how you and your family handle difficult situations. What do you want them to learn? Write what you want your children to learn and refer to it often:

You and your children will be learning many lessons during your journey toward wellness. Here are some of them:
It is permissible to talk about cancer.
The expectation is that you and they can handle whatever happens.
Since your children may become flooded with feelings, you can teach them how to regulate those feelings by talking and saying calming statements, learning relaxation responses like deep breathing, hugging (hugging actually calms and contributes biochemically to inhibiting tears), just like you are learning from this workbook and CD.
They should not be ashamed of cancer or their own distress about it.
They and their family can figure out effective coping skills to handle difficult situations.
Their family is there for support and they can count on their family to be honest.
They are deeply loved always, from wherever you are.

These are important life lessons. These are important messages you can start telling your child right now.
Write other lessons you want to teach your children. Let these lessons be your guide. Make them part of your conversations with your children.

_____
_____
_____
_____
_____

What to Tell Elderly Parents

My patients often ask me how to break the news to their elderly parents. Again, this is not easy. First is the issue of whether or not to tell. If your parents are mentally competent and physically well enough, then you should tell them. If they are not mentally competent, or are suffering through a life-threatening or debilitating illness of their own, then I suggest you talk to other family members, your parent's physician, and a therapist who specializes in the elderly population about whether or not to tell them.

It is always preferable to tell the truth, of course. But sometimes aging and fragile parents can't handle the whole truth and you need to tell a part of the truth. The sorrow, fear, and anxiety might be too much to handle because they no longer have the physical, emotional, and spiritual resources that they once had. But you will need to figure out something to tell them because chances are high something will change and they will notice a difference in you and in your routine. You might not be able to visit as often or do caretaking tasks like you did. They will notice that you might be tired from your treatments, or that you have lost your hair or that your body has changed in some way. When you can, please be honest. Discuss with others who know your parents and who know the special needs of the elderly the best way to help your parents through your illness.

Just like telling your children was so difficult because of your desire to protect them from hardship, telling your elderly parents will be difficult for the same reason. And there may be an added sorrow. Your parents may be too old to help take care of you now, and to many of my patients, this is a painful loss. Many adults with cancer have the inner desire, "I want my Mommy now. I want my Daddy now". They want someone to step in and make it all better. Some face the loss that they never had a mommy or daddy who was a good caretaker. Others had good mommies or daddies, but their ability to nurture is now impaired. For those whose parents have died, cancer may bring renewed grief. Some people believe in a spiritual life after death. If that is your belief, then you can invite the comforting spirits of your parents to be with you now.

If grief bubbles up for you, remind yourself that you are on a journey learning how to take good care of yourself with the support of others. For every moving on, there is a loss. Let yourself feel it, take in a deep breath, and tell yourself you are doing what you need to do to get well.

Talking with Your Friends

Decide which friends you want to tell. Tell them as soon as you can and tell them the truth. Friends often want to help. Tell them what they can do for you. Tell them how often you want to be called. Tell them if you need rides to treatments. Tell them if you would like company during chemotherapy. Tell them if you need some cooked meals, an errand run, or help driving carpool. Tell them if they can make phone calls for you. Tell them if you want to watch a video with them. And tell them when you want to be alone.

My point is that you are in charge of how you will handle your journey to wellness. *It is your responsibility to let others know what you need from them.* I know this can be easy to say and hard to do. It helps to say "I do need help. These are the things I need help with. What would you feel comfortable doing?...thank you."

*   *   *   *

List helpful friends:

_____

_____

_____

_____

_____

Just like the other people in your life, your friends will have reactions to you. Their reactions will be similar to everyone else's, depending on how close they are to you. They will also have an identification reaction that may be scary for them, because if cancer could happen to you at your age, it could happen to them, too. If you feel up to talking about this with them, that's fine. But it's also fine to not process this with your friends. Do whatever is best for you. Your friends can talk to other people about their anxieties. You don't have to take care of them now. Your priority is to take care of you. Your taking good care of yourself is a gift and an example to them, just like their helping you is their gift to you.

Talking with Business Associates

It is up to you who to tell and what to tell at work. Of course, if your treatments mean that you'll miss some work, then you'll need to discuss your situation with your boss or your business partners and make the best arrangements that you can. After that, talk to whomever will be affected by your changes. It has been the experience of my patients that people find out anyway. Even those who decided not to tell anyone at work, find they get phone calls of caring and concern from coworkers they haven't seen for years who heard the news though the grapevine. Generally, after initial reluctance about telling people, they were glad to receive the kind words, good wishes, and prayers.

As Soon as Possible and as Much as Possible, Get On with Your Life

Being told to get on with your life can be maddening. But it helps. As much as you can, keep the rituals and routines of your life the same as before. There is so much comfort in familiar habits, in the little details of life. Just like I told you to keep details and rituals the same for children, it's important that you do that for yourself. It is also important to develop some new rituals that will become comforting as they turn into old habits.

"I remember how bitterly I resented those who blithely suggested that I get on with my usual activities....There is some sort of quiet rebuilding going on, as if the infrastructure of my spirit is being shored up" (Musa Mayer, Examining Myself).

*   *   *   *

Comforting rituals

_____

_____

_____

_____

_____

Humor

Laughter helps. It relaxes you and boosts your immune system. It decreases stress, and there is even some evidence that it increases blood levels of antibodies that help fight bacteria and viruses. Some studies have linked laughter with reduced pain and pain tolerance. It certainly improves your mood, takes your mind off distress, and helps you feel connected to others.

"Joy is what recharges you. It helps and rejuvenates you for whatever fight you have ahead.
Just like scheduling medical appointments, it's important to schedule times to recharge the joy"
(Peggy Rios, Ph.D. Program Director, The Cancer Support Community of Greater Miami, Miami, FL).

"Humor is the great thing, the saving thing. The minute it crops up, all our irritations and resentments slip away and a sunny spirit takes their place" (Mark Twain).

"Laughter gives us distance. It allows us to step back from an event, deal with it, and then move on"
(Bob Newhart).

"Always laugh if you can. It is cheap medicine" (Lord Byron).

"I made the joyous discovery that ten minutes of genuine belly laughter had anesthetic effect and would give me at least two hours of pain-free sleep" (Norman Cousins, Anatomy of an Illness).

*   *   *   *

What makes you smile and laugh? Make a list. There are times you may forget what makes you laugh and it helps to have a list ready. You may want to include movies, children, grandchildren, pets, comedians, TV shows, activities.

_____

_____

_____

_____

_____

Letting Go of Anger

"Holding onto anger is like grasping a hot coal with the intent of throwing it at someone else; you are the one getting burned" (Buddha).

Anger is disconnecting. This chapter, in fact this whole book, is about finding connections during a time in your life that can be very disconnecting.

Recognize any anger that you have, and then let it go. People often get angry at God, themselves, family members, doctors, the world. Yours might be a direct anger, or it might emerge as a general irritability. It may also get worse when you are tired, achy, or nauseas. It is normal to have some anger when dealing with cancer. If your anger lasts for a month, is persistent, and is interfering with your ability to function and have satisfying relationships, please get help from your support group or seek individual counseling. Let your anger energize you, and then let it go.

Art

Why Amy Paints
She says, "It helps to put it out there,"
Whatever IT is that we need to put outside of us
Because it takes up too much room inside.
 (Claudia W. Reder, Poet)

Art can help. Sometimes it's hard to express feelings and experiences in words. That makes it harder to connect with other people, and harder to connect with yourself. Art is a wonderful way to express yourself and connect deep within and offer it as a connection to others. There are many mediums: paint, clay, cut-outs, pictures, photography, and more. Find an art class, an art therapist, draw with friends, buy some art paper and just see what happens. You don't have to be a talented artist. This art is not to be evaluated as good or bad. Like your feelings, your art just *is*.

Remember Chapter 2. I told you that you need to know your feelings because they are such a valuable source of information. Well, art can help you understand this information. It can be a bridge to inside.

Many of my patients find drawing mandalas interesting and helpful. Mandalas are graphic circles divided into sections and are used as instruments of meditation. The word is Sanskrit for circle, and is thought of as a representation of the universe. Your mandala can be your own universe. By mentally entering, or thinking about your mandala, your attention will be eventually drawn to the center. There are many ways to do mandalas. Here's a suggestion:

*   *   *   *

Mandala exercise: draw a circle, divide the circle into three parts. In one part, draw something that represents what you want for your body. In another section, draw what you want for your mind, and in the last section, draw what you want for your spirit. Then in the middle, draw what connects them. Take your time. Don't judge what you are doing. Just let it happen. When you finish, put it away. After three to seven days, take it out and write what you understand from your drawing. This can be repeated because what you want for yourself may change. If you wish, you can share your drawing with other people.

What did you draw in each section?
Which was the hardest section to draw?
Which was the easiest?
What does that mean to you?
Are all the sections the same size?
How did you connect the three parts?

Some people like to color mandalas that are already in printed designs. You can find coloring books of mandalas and you can find websites on the internet with selections of mandala designs you can easily print out. Then, you let your attention focus on the design, choose your color medium, and begin. People find that coloring in the repetitive, circular movement is very comforting. As their attention is naturally drawn to the center, they enter a meditative state.

Writing
Many of my patients write daily or weekly journals, write poetry, or write their thoughts and feelings only occasionally. You may find this helpful too. You may want to read what you write often, or you may find that you want to put it away and not look at it for a long time

because you're tired of dealing with cancer. That's fine, too. Just know that writing is another way of connecting to yourself and to others.

This chapter has been about connections. Connections are the relationships that help you grow. They offer you the energy to do what you have to do, the support to take care of yourself, and the hope to move forward in your fight against cancer.

CHAPTER 6

Taking Charge

Spirituality

Many People Turn to Spirituality in Times of Need

And I will take the spirit which is upon thee, and will put it upon them; and they shall bear the burden of the people with thee, that thou bear it not thyself alone
  (Numbers 11:17).

Ask, and it shall be given you; seek, and ye shall find; knock and it shall be opened unto you:
For everyone that asketh receiveth; and he that seeketh findeth; and to him that knocheth it shall be opened
  (Matthew 7:7).

"May the Force be with you" (George W. Lucas, Jr. Star Wars).

National surveys consistently support the idea that religion and spirituality are important to most of us. More than 90% of adults express a belief in God, and slightly more than 70% of those surveyed identified religion as one of the most important influences in their lives. (Gallup GH: Religion In America 1996: Will the Vitality of the Church Be the Surprise of the 21st Century?. Princeton, NJ: Princeton Religion Research Center, 1996.)Research indicates that patients commonly rely on spirituality and religion to help them deal with serious physical illnesses. A survey of hospital inpatients found that 77% of patients reported that physicians should take patients' spiritual needs into consideration, and 37% wanted physicians to address religious beliefs more frequently. (King DE, Bushwick B: Beliefs and attitudes of hospital inpatients about faith healing and prayer. J Fam Pract 39 (4): 349-52, 1994.)

Religion and Spirituality

Some people feel that the difference between religion and spirituality is important. Other people feel they refer to the same experience and practice. Your belief is personal. Whether or not there is a distinction for you depends on your personal beliefs and your expression of them.

Religion generally refers to a specific set of beliefs and rituals that are associated in an organized way. Spirituality generally refers to the experience of a set of beliefs that engages a person in feelings of connectedness to him or herself, the community, and/or nature and the universe. Some people think of themselves as religious but not spiritual, some people think of themselves as spiritual but not religious. Others say that they are both. All these categories can be beneficial to your health. My patients who choose to find comfort in their religion and spirituality seem to be looking for deeper connection and meaning in their lives.

Religion and Spirituality Have a Positive Effect on Quality of Life and Health

Scientific research validates that a rich spiritual life is a powerful influence on our wellness. Some studies show that praying can help improve the immune system, improve cardiac function, and reduce stress, worry, and anxiety.

Larry Dossey, in his several excellent books, talks about the local and nonlocal mind. We all know about our local mind: it's the one inside our heads. He talks about the evidence for a nonlocal mind, or a collective unconscious, a universal energy to which we are all connected. When we pray, he says, we are communicating through the nonlocal mind.

How Do You Define Your Religiosity and Spirituality?

- Faith is an individual experience.

- Some people look for a connection to themselves.

- Some people look for a connection to other people.

- Some people look for a connection to nature and the beauty and orderliness of the world.

- Some people look for a connection to God.

- Some people turn to a Higher Power.

- Some people look for a connection to the Universe

- Some people look for a mutuality of power.

- Some strive to be better people.

"...when I say spiritual I mean basic human good qualities. These are: human affection, a sense of involvement, honesty, discipline and human intelligence properly guided by

good motivation. We have all these qualities from birth; they do not come to us later in our lives" (His Holiness The Dalai Lama).

Explore your own religious and spiritual beliefs with the questionnaire below.

Spirituality Questionnaire

This questionnaire grew out of my many conversations with patients and friends. These are the kinds of questions about which they thought and wanted to talk. You may find them helpful too. You can answer them in order, or you can choose any order. You can choose one question, or you can choose several at a time.

<u>Questionnaire</u>
How do you define "religion"?
How do you define "spirituality"?
Did you grow up in an organized religion?
What is your earliest memory about religion?
Was it a positive experience for you?
What is your earliest memory about spiritual things?
What were your grandparents beliefs?
What are your mother's beliefs?
What are your father's beliefs?
What are your impressions about how your mother and father dealt with their beliefs as a couple?
What were the family expectations for you with regard to religion or spirituality?
Do you believe in God?
What is your concept of God?
Is there a purpose to life?
Is it necessary to connect with others?
Do you have to be part of a greater community to experience your concept of God?
What comforts you when you are in pain, scared, or feeling alone?
Is your spirit the same as your soul?
Do you have faith?
What does it mean to you "to have faith"?
Do you believe that your faith can heal your body?
Do you believe your faith can heal your mind?
Do you believe your faith can heal your spirit?

Do you believe that nourishing your spirit benefits your mind and body?
How does being religious help you?
How does being spiritual help you?
Are you intuitive?
Do your religious or spiritual beliefs help you deal with loss?
Name two people whom you most admire. Why do you admire them?
Do you ever feel "connected" to people? How does this feel for you?
Do you ever feel "connected" to nature? How does this feel for you?
Do you ever feel "connected" to something greater than yourself? How does this feel for you?
What do I fear the most?
What makes me the saddest?
What comforts me?
What brings me joy?
Is gratefulness an important concept to you?
Are you a grateful person?
What are you grateful for?
Is forgiveness an important concept to you?
Are you a forgiving person?
Do you pray?
Do you think God or your concept of God, hears or answers prayers?
My daily prayer is:

_____
_____
_____
_____
_____

What are your beliefs about:

- Life

- Death

- What happens after someone dies

- People

- The Universe

- God

- How do you connect with your concept of God?

- Prayer
- Rituals
- Angels
- Spirits
- Soul
- Energy

*   *   *   *

Please discuss the questionnaire with others. Talk about it with your family and colleagues at work. Bring it to your support group, talk about it with friends, take it to your church, synagogue, mosque or any religious/spiritual meeting place. Talking with others helps you express your feelings and thoughts. Hearing others' beliefs will help you explore your own. Conversations about your religious and spiritual beliefs deepen your own understanding of yourself and connect you to others in a deeply personal way. Feel free to add your own questions and answers.

Many cancer patients find that their religious and spiritual beliefs deepen and change as they work toward recovery. When they are in remission, they continue to explore their faith. Many years later, they are still growing and connecting with their faith.

Ways to Experience Spiritual Growth

"Just as the hand, held before the eye, can hide the tallest mountain, so the routine of everyday life can keep us from seeing the vast radiance and the secret wonders that fill the world" (Chasidic, 18ᵗʰ Century, from Gates of Repentance, The New Union Prayer Book).

To experience your personal spiritual growth, it helps to be open to whatever paths you wish to explore. Here us a wonderful meditation exercise that creates the experience of openness and receptivity so that you can discover what spirituality is like for you.

*   *   *   *

Rosebud Meditation
By Holly W. Schwartztol, Ph.D.

Gently close your eyes. Take in a deep breath and slowly, slowly release the breath. Now, as you bring your awareness to the center of your chest, imagine that there is a tiny rosebud. And, I don't know what color you might choose for your rosebud. It might be red or yellow or pink or white or even a combination of colors, it doesn't matter. Just allow the rosebud to take form.

Now, imagine that golden sunlight is shining on your rosebud....and as that happens, notice that your rosebud is opening petal ...by petal... by petal... until it blossoms into a full blown rose. Then, softly bring your awareness back into the room and gently open your eyes.

Here are some ways that my patients have used to discover their religious and spiritual paths.

- Make a commitment to cultivate your personal faith.
- *"I believe in a benevolent spirit that animates the universe" (Francis L. Carter)*
- Join a support group.
- Reach out for spiritual allies.
- Join an organized religion.
- Practice rituals of organized religion.
- Create your own rituals.
- *"There is no need to go to India or anywhere else to find peace. You will find that deep place of silence right in your room, your garden or even your bathtub" (Elizabeth Kubler-Ross)*
- Join a prayer group.
- Find a psychic, intuitive or medium.
- Pray with trusted members of your healthcare team.
- Meditate.
- Find relaxation techniques you like.
- Practice forgiveness.
- *"Life is an adventure in forgiveness" (Norman Cousins).*
- *"Always forgive your enemies; nothing annoys them so much" (Oscar Wilde).*
- Make a private quiet time and pray.
- Connect with nature.
- *"I believe in God, only I spell it Nature" (Frank Lloyd Wright).*

- *"Raising things up is jolly nice" (John Brooks on gardening on NPR, The Diane Rheem show 10/31/03)*

- Plan quiet times.

- *"Stop leaving and you will arrive. Stop searching and you will see. Stop running away and you will be found" (Lao Tzu).*

- Be kind to yourself.

- Practice kindness to others: do good deeds and help others.

- *"When we feel love and kindness toward others, it not only makes others feel loved and cared for, but it helps us also to develop inner happiness and peace" (His Holiness The Dalai Lama).*

- Practice self-exploration: connecting to yourself opens the window to connecting with others, which opens the door to connecting with the Universe.

- Keep a wonderful moments diary.

- Give thanks every day.

- *"Happiness makes up in height for what it lacks in length" (Robert Frost).*

- **Be the best person you can be.**

- *"Lead your life so you wouldn't be ashamed to sell the family parrot to the town gossip" (Will Rogers).*

Your spiritual path will unfold over time. It's a process. There is no end, no "there" there. It's a process of personal growth and discovery that offers comfort, joy, and peace. I know that you have started on your path because you're reading this chapter. You are not alone on your journey. Reach out for support in finding your way (see chapter 5). There's lots of support for you. Many patients say that their spiritual growth is the gift of having cancer because their lives are enriched and more meaningful. This can happen for you. You're doing very, very well, and you're doing your best.

CHAPTER 7

Taking Charge

Taking Action: My Plan

"Nothing contributes so much to tranquilizing the mind as a steady purpose – a point on which the soul may fix its intellectual eye" (Mary Wollstonecraft Shelley).

Making Decisions

"Once you make a decision, the universe conspires to make it happen" (Ralph Waldo Emerson).

You have a lot of decisions to make, a lot of people to talk to, treatments to learn about, lifestyle changes to make, family issues to deal with, and…well, the list goes on and on. At times, most of my patients feel overwhelmed. It helps to create a plan of action that you write down on paper or input in your computer to feel organized about what you're doing and where you're heading. Research shows that people who write things down are more likely to get them done. Managing your time in this way will relieve stress and help you feel calmer because you will feel more in control—*that you have personally taken charge of your fight against cancer.*

Identify Your Target, Set Your Intention, and Do What you Need To Do
Creating goals and setting priorities

First, make a list of everything you think you have to do. Just put it on paper in whatever order it comes up. Take the time you need to do this. It always takes more than one sitting. Remember that this is a "live list." It will change as your needs change. Then put it aside for a little while.

Now, I'd like you to remember some of our earlier discussions about how fighting cancer involves your *body, mind, and spirit*. I told you that you need to attend to all three, and that as you take care of each one, you will positively affect the other two. For example, as you take care of your mind by practicing positive thinking skills, your body will be more relaxed, and you'll be more open to connecting to your spiritual beliefs. Mind, body, and spirit are three equally important, interrelated aspects of your being. Actually, together, they form a seamless web. It's just for purposes of getting organized to take care of ourselves that we divide them into separate parts. Throughout this book, you've been learning how to take care of each part.

Your goals are what you want to accomplish. They are your desired results. They are your *targets* for fighting cancer. You achieve them by setting your intention, or focus, on them— by purposely devising a course of action. Then, you do something towards your targets everyday. For example, your long range goal might be to take a vacation. That's your target. Short range goals, your *intentions,* to get to your target might be to explore vacation places, how much they cost, discovering if you want an adventure week or a relaxing sit-on-the-beach week, finding out how long you can take off from work, etc. Your *do* list is your "things to do today" list, which might be to call the airlines, talk to a travel agent, talk to friends about where they have traveled, make a reservation, etc.

You see, once you identify your targets, you can set your intention to do what needs to be done to achieve your desired results. I know you do this already in many aspects of your life. Even going to the grocery store involves this process.

Target: get food in the house.

Intention: figure out when I can go, which store I will go to, how much money is in my budget this week.

Do today: check cabinets and refrigerator, make a list, mark my calendar for time to go.

The same process you already use to achieve the big and small targets in your life, I want you to use here. But because cancer is more complicated, you need to be more organized. Here is what I suggest. Get out that big list you prepared earlier. It will be a handy reference.

You have three main targets to reach: body, mind, and spirit. What do you want for each?

Get a wide piece of paper, perhaps 9" x 18". If this size is not readily available, you can tape together two 8 ½" x 11"'s. Across the top put your three main goals or targets. It may look like this:

Targets
Body
To be cancer-free

Mind
To focus my mind to aid my body and sustain my spirit in getting well

Spirit
To be open to deeper connections to myself, others, and my beliefs about the Universe

Intentions
Body
Find the best doctors
Find out about clinical trials
Find out about nutrition
Find out about exercise

Mind
Become calmer and more relaxed
Find out about positive thinking skills
Learn how to get motivated and focused
Find cancer survivors and learn from them

Spirit
Explore values: what is really important to me
Find support group
Meditate
Explore how to connect better with my family

Do Today
Body
Write list of questions to ask my doctor
Go to doctor's appointment
Attend yoga class
Take nap at 3:00 p.m.

Mind
Listen to *Fighting Cancer*
Create my personal affirmations

Practice my affirmations
Ask a cancer survivor what she said to herself to stay positively focused on getting well

Spirit
Attend support group
Attend a worship service
Do a good deed for the day
Talk with my best friend

As you can see, the lists overlap. For example, you may decide to put support group in the "Mind" column. Or, you may put *Fighting Cancer* in your "Spiritual" column. There are no absolute rules. What matters is that you get your list right for you.

- write down your targets

- write down your intentions

- write down your lists of things to do today and

- —and most important of all—

- ***Do something towards your targets everyday.***

"Planning is bringing the future into the present so you can do something about it now" (Alan Lakein, How to Get Control of Your Time and Your Life).

Then you will be taking the best care of yourself in as *balanced* a way as you can. You'll feel better, you'll feel more in control, and you'll have a written record of what you have done, where you are now, and where you're headed. You know that old saying, "ready, set, go!" *Identify your target, set your intention, and do what you need to do – every day.*

Now you are working in an organized way on your list of everything you need and want to do. You are working on prioritizing your list. You understand that over time your *targets* may change, your *intentions* for achieving your targets will change as you progress, and certainly your *do today* list will change daily.

If you are having trouble prioritizing your lists, it will help to ask yourself two important questions about each item:
What will happen if I do this now?
What will happen if I don't do this now?
You'll quickly begin to discover which items are the most important for you today.

For example, finding out what treatments are available may be more important than tending your garden right now. Listening to *Fighting Cancer* first thing in the morning so you can motivate and calm yourself may be more important than writing an update letter for friends. Calling doctors' offices to set up appointments may be more important than calling some friends. Check priorities carefully and often. They will change as your needs change. Keep them flexible.

Balancing your needs and things to do may be a challenge some days. Be sure to include dealing with pain, fatigue, and mush-brain in your plans. Talk to your healthcare team about what treatments are available to help if you're experiencing fatigue and/or mush-brain. Talk to cancer survivors to find out how they handled these problems. Remember, lots of people have and are going through what you are experiencing. Let them share with you what they know, and you can share with them what you are learning.

You may want to choose a system to organize your targets. Spend some time exploring what is available. Choose a system that is easy to use, helps you clarify what you need to do, has room for targets, intentions, and what you need to do today. Here are efficient examples of what of my patients have used to help them feel in control of their time and lives.

- Personal computer
- Big paper
- Hand held computer organizers, e.g. Balckberry, Iphone, etc,
- Planner Pad (plannerpads.com)
- Cancer Support Community organization materials (cancersupportcommunity.org, this has useful, specific charts for things like tracking symptoms)
- Spending time at an office supply store to see what is the latest and best for you
- Large dry erase board

As you work on your lists of targets, intentions, and what to do today, your tasks and desires will become clearer and clearer. In addition to *doing* the tasks you need to do, you can give your intentions and targets to the back of your mind, to your unconscious mind. Sometimes, your unconscious mind will find answers that your conscious mind is not aware of yet. Have you ever struggled with a problem and just couldn't figure out a solution? Then, you "forgot" about it, went to do something else, and then perhaps the next day the solution popped into your mind. That's your unconscious mind at work. Let it help you now.

*　　*　　*　　*

Find a comfortable place to sit for just a few minutes. One at a time, let a picture form in your mind of each of your targets. In your creative mind's eye, visualize giving your targets to the back of your mind. You may see yourself handing a special file into a beautiful filing cabinet, or you may see a bubble filled with gorgeous colors moving into the back of your head, or it may be a feeling that you experience, or a thought that you say to yourself, such as "I am giving the target of picturing myself cancer-free to the back of my unconscious mind". Then, go do something else.

That's it. It's that simple. Do this once a week, more or less, as you need it. Your unconscious mind is concrete and it likes specific instructions. It's a powerful inner resource for you.

As you give focus and attention to what you need to do, you'll use both your knowledge and your intuition. You already have a lot of knowledge, which is the information you are learning through your experience, doctors, healthcare team, reading, talking to others, internet searches, and other sources. Intuition is the information you get from sources that don't always feel rational. It is the decision-making method that you use unconsciously. It's a rapid and creative process. It's the process you use when you say things like "I know it in my gut," or "I know it's the right thing to do." As you make your treatment plans, you'll be using both kinds of decision making processes.

Some of my patients find the following exercise calming and useful when they have gathered a lot of knowledge and want to check in with themselves to decide a plan of action. It's a widely used exercise called

*　　*　　*　　*

The Inner Advisor Imagery Exercise

Breathe in slowly, and exhale slowly. Do this a few times. Close your eyes when you're ready. That's right. Now, picture yourself in a lovely, peaceful, soothing place. Maybe you're at a beach, in a meadow, lying on your bed, in a park…wherever you are, as long as you feel very comfortable, it's a good choice for you. Find a place to sit, or walk slowly if you prefer. Look around at what is there, smell any fragrances and aromas, listen to the sounds, touch what is near you, and notice any pleasant taste in your mouth. Let yourself become aware of what it's like to be there. That's right. Take a few moments to enjoy the relaxation, the peace, and the comfort.

Now, whenever you're ready, invite your inner advisor to join you. Your inner advisor might take the form of a wise old man or woman, an animal, a ball of softly glowing light, or some other form. Whatever form it takes is fine, as long as it feels wise, compassionate, safe, and helpful to you.

Now, ask your inner advisor the question you need answered…..give yourself plenty of time to receive the answer in what ever form it's given to you. You may receive your answer in words, in a symbol, a feeling, or some other form of communication. You may understand what the answer means, or you may not understand right now. Either way is fine. Just be open to receiving whatever comes to you. You may not understand the communication right away. Sometimes, a week later, people find they're driving somewhere and suddenly the meaning of the communication becomes clear. I want you to know that whatever is happening for you in this exercise, you are doing very well. Let this process unfold and allow your knowledge and intuition to work together for you.

Write down your experience doing this exercise so you can remember it for use now or later.

_____

_____

_____

_____

_____

Tips:

- Plan in plenty of rest times.

- Get to know your best times of the day and how you want to use them.

- Be flexible with your schedule.

- Be kind and forgiving to yourself if you don't get everything done. (Prioritizing helps with this. When you can't get to everything, you'll know you've done the most important things first)

- *You come first, so learn to say no to others.*

Visualize Your Targets

"Go confidently in the direction of your dreams. Live the life you have imagined" (Henry David Thoreau).

*   *   *   *

Creating a Treasure Map

A treasure map is a visual representation of your targets and intentions. It's a visual affirmation, a visual expression of the things you want for yourself and what you want in your life. You literally create a picture of your future and display it where you'll see it often. It's based on the ideas of Shakti Gawain in her 1978 book, Creative Visualization.

Think about how you want to display your future. Some people use a poster board, some people create dioramas, picture books in loose leaf format, a mobile, or anything that comes to mind for you is fine, as long as you can put it where you'll see it often.

Cut out pictures from magazines, draw pictures, use photos, or paint what you would like to have in your life. Cut out or write words or phrases. Perhaps you'll make a collage. Or maybe you'll divide a poster board into three parts representing your body, mind, and spirit; or maybe you'll divide it into five parts and have health, nutrition, marriage, family, and travel. You think about what is important to you, and your way to organize will emerge.

Always present what you want for your future in a positive way. For example, do not include "less stress", for then you would have to include a representation of stress. Instead, you could put "more calmness", and include a representation of what is calming for you.

Put something that represents you in the middle. It could be a photo, your name, or a symbol with which you identify.

Be creative. It's your future.

I hope that I have been able to pass on to you what I have learned from so many people. I hope that this information eases your recovery and I sincerely and heartily wish you well on your journey.

Resources

"As the shock of my diagnosis began to wear off, and as I commenced treatment and began to accept the fact that I was and would continue to be living with cancer, I felt the need for contact with others who were experiencing the same things, both phsycally and psychologically, as I. Eventually I did discover that there are many helpers out there" (Marcia H. Kenward).

There are many resources available in your community and on the internet. According to Consumer Reports On Health, October, 2004, there are questions to consider for safe surfing:
What is the site's intent? Reputable sites clearly state their purpose.
Who owns and operates the site? Be wary of sites tied to specific products. Check the "Contact Us" section, reputable organizations will fully disclose their contact information.
What are the sites' privacy policies? Be especially careful if you are entering health or credit card information.
What is the source of the information cited? Reference, data, and credentials should be available.
How often is the site updated?

This is a list to help you get started. It is not a comprehensive list.

General Cancer Information

National Cancer Institute (NCI): www.cancer.gov

Tel. 800.422.6237

NCI offers a guide for patients seeking a doctor or treatment center for cancer. On the web, at http://cis.nci.nih.gov/fact/7_47.htm, the guide includes advice and numerous resources for finding a specialist, getting a second opinion, choosing a treatment, and useful links.

American Cancer Society: www.cancer.org

National Library of Medicine
MedlinePlus Health Information: www.nlm.nih.gov/medlineplus

Information about clinical trials

National Cancer Institute: www.cancer.gov/trials
National Institutes of Health: www.clincialtrials.gov/
Centerwatch: www.centerwatch.com/patient/trials.html

Finding professional psychological help

Ask your oncologist for referrals
Local psychological association
Local psychiatric association
Local mental health association
Nearby colleges and universities have counseling centers
Hospitals often have support groups and other helpful resources

Breast Cancer

Susan G. Komen Breast Cancer Foundation: www.komen.org
Breast cancer information, research, and community, with 100 local affiliates.
National Breast Cancer Coalition: www.stopbreastcancer.org
Y-Me: www.y-me.org
More support: www.breastcancer.org,

Pain

American Pain Foundation: www.painfoundatoin.org
Tel. 888.615.7246
Offers a free notebook to help you track your pain experience so you can provide the information to your healthcare team

Complementary and Alternative Medicine

National Center for Complementary and Alternative Medicine (NCCAM) Clearinghouse
www.nccam.nih.gov
Tel. 888.644.6226
Complementary and Alternative Medicine on PubMed

www.nim.nih.gov/nccam/camonpubmed.html
Food and Drug Administration
www.fda.gov
The Cancer Support Community
www.cancersupportcommunity.org
The Cancer Support Community is a national non-profit organization dedicated to providing free emotional, support, education, and hope for people with cancer and their loved ones. They have facilities nationwide, and online support groups.

Support

The Cancer Support Community (see above)

CancerCare: www.cancercare.org

A nonprofit agency that helps people with cancer, families, and friends cope with the impact of the disease

National Coalition for cancer survivorship: www.cansearch.org

La Liga Contra el Cancer: 305.856.4915

Offers cancer information and support in Spanish

More resources: www.livestrong.org/Get-Help/Find-More-Resources

Magazine

CURE (Cancer Updates, Research, & Education), a magazine for cancer patients and their caregivers

www.curetoday.com

To Translate Medical Language Into Words You Can Understand

Medical Library Association: www.mlanet.org/resources/medspeak/

For common medical terms

National Library of Medicine: www.medlinepluc.gov

For a comprehensive database of information

Merck Manual of Health Information: www.merck.com/mrkshared/manual_home2home.jsp

For information about diseases, procedures, and other health issues

American Association for Clinical Chemistry: www.labtestinline.org

For information about lab tests and terminology

The Guided Imagery Collection

available at

www.drscarter.com

and for download at Itunes

RELAXING MEDITATIONS FOR HEALTH AND HEALING
With Dr. Stephanie R. Carter

Listen to relaxing imagery with Dr. Carter's soothing voice over calming, classical music. Each CD has a different focus, depending on your needs.

FIGHTING CANCER

This CD is healing visual imagery and soothing music designed to help you relax, reduce anxiety and pain, boost your immune system, and to motivate you to fight cancer. It is most effective when used with *Taking Charge of Fighting Cancer, an easy to use workbook* by Dr. Carter.

CREATE YOUR UNIQUE RELAXING PLACE

This CD is for you to use anytime you want to relax and let go of all your tension and worries. It is for you when you want to relieve pain, calm your thoughts and sleep restfully. It can be used by itself, or with any of the other CDs, because it is helpful for any situation.

FOR YOUR SURGERY
BEFORE, DURING, AND AFTER

This CD is designed to help you during your entire surgical experience. It is easy to use.

Listen as many times as you can before surgery.

Listen during surgery. Tell your surgeon that you would like to listen during surgery. Most surgeons welcome anything that is safe and helpful, so he/she will welcome this too. Be sure to get a CD player and learn how to set it for continuous play to that the exercise will repeat over and over again during the whole time of your surgery. Get earphones so that you can listen without distracting your surgical team. Remember to get fresh batteries for you CD player.

Listen after surgery, during your recovery, as many times as you wish. The suggestions for healing are healthy and positive for both your mind and body.

APPRECIATING

This CD is designed to enhance spirituality. It promotes positive thinking and enhances feelings of well-being. You are guided to draw strength from your past as you look forward to your future. You remember positive people from your past and you reintroduce their love and support into your life now, as you prepare for the future.

CALMING YOUR CHILD NIGHT AND DAY

Teach your child how to use his or her imagination to relax and find comfort any time of the day or night, how to calm down from a tantrum, how to let go of fears and worries, and how to fall peacefully asleep.

There are two tracks. The first is a fun, interactive and soothing adventure with playful, gentle sound effects.

The second includes Loving Thoughts, which are affirmations every child needs to hear.